ROCKINGHAM COLLEGE
LIBRARY
5815

Bereavement and grief
Supporting older people through loss

D0306393

Bereavement and grief
Supporting older people through loss

Steve Scrutton
CQSW, BSc (Econ), MA, Cert Ed, Dip Ed

Operational Social Work Manager, Northamptonshire

Edward Arnold
A member of the Hodder Headline Group
LONDON   SYDNEY   AUCKLAND

5 8 1 5
6·6·95

First published in Great Britain 1995 by
Edward Arnold, a division of Hodder Headline PLC,
338 Euston Road, London NW1 3BH

Co-published with Age Concern England,
Astral House, 1268 London Road, London SW16 4EJ

© 1995 Steve Scrutton

All rights reserved. No part of this publication may be reproduced or
transmitted in any form or by any means, electronically or mechanically,
including photocopying, recording or any information storage or retrieval
system, without either prior permission in writing from the publisher or a
licence permitting restricted copying. In the United Kingdom such licences
are issued by the Copyright Licensing Agency: 90 Tottenham Court Road,
London W1P 9HE.

Whilst the advice and information in this book is believed to be true and
accurate at the date of going to press, neither the author nor the publisher
can accept any legal responsibility or liability for any errors or omissions
that may be made.

British Library Cataloguing in Publication Data
A catalogue record for this book is available from the British Library

ISBN 0 340 60482 4

1 2 3 4 5   95 96 97 98 99

Typeset in 10/12 pt Palatino by GreenGate Publishing Services, Tonbridge, Kent
Printed and bound in Great Britain by J W Arrowsmith Ltd, Bristol

Contents

Introduction

The experience of loss in older age

Loss is an experience common to people of all ages. Loss in older age, however, often assumes a particular piquancy because of the familiar assumption, frequently incorrect, that loss becomes increasingly irreplaceable with advancing age, and that it becomes harder to recover from the emotional distress that can result from loss.

Loss restricts us all, and dealing with the grief caused to older people can be extremely difficult. The older individual will often require considerable assistance to come to terms with what has happened, especially when systems of support have been considerably reduced.

The task of support primarily falls upon a few relatives and close friends who can feel unprepared to face such a task. Sometimes professional assistance is inadequate, sparse or even non-existent, with the result that well-intentioned but unprepared carers are left with the problem of coping on their own in dealing with the trauma.

Age Concern, England, have been aware of the situation for some time, and this book is the result of the identification of the need for an uncomplicated, straightforward text to support them in their task.

1 Bereavement, older age and ageism

Bereavement, loss, grief and mourning

The popular definition of bereavement concerns the loss through death of someone to whom there has been a strong, loving attachment. The experience is widely recognised as one of the most severe traumas that people have to cope with in life, requiring that the individual comes to terms with the fundamental changes that loss has brought about, changes that often involve a revolution in an entire lifestyle which, until recently, was taken for granted.

The process of forming close personal attachments begins in childhood. The theory of attachment (Bowlby, 1980) seeks to explain why people make strong bonds of affection with other people, the essential goal being to maintain stability in life. The value of attachment is best illustrated in child development, when children begin to leave the 'attachment figures', usually parents, for increasing periods of time in order to explore the world, but do so safe in the knowledge that they can always return home for the protection and reassurance they require.

The impact of bereavement on attachment and the stability and certainty it harbours, can be devastating. Significant aspects of life, previously considered of fundamental importance, will have been irretrievably lost. The individual can feel entirely alone and abandoned. Life can appear unbearably painful, incomplete, and disorienting. When important attachments are threatened, broken, or irrevocably lost, it creates intense emotional anxiety and acute social difficulties, the combination of which requires a major life-readjustment to ensure personal survival.

It is vital to realise that the importance of attachment, and the impact of bereavement, do not decline with age. The loss of significant, long-standing relationships is as damaging to the older individual as the loss of a parent in childhood, but unfortunately, the gravity of such losses in older age is not always fully recognised. Bereavement can lead to:

- feelings of unfairness, anger and rage
- feelings of guilt, and personal responsibility for what has occurred

- changed feelings about personal worth, values, and identity
- a changed awareness and recognition of the ageing process, and personal mortality
- the undermining of a sense of well-being, often giving rise to physical and mental illness
- feelings of acute anxiety, and fears about the future.

Bereavement can so seriously affect the daily functioning of the individual that it is sometimes perceived to be, and is treated as, an illness. Engel (1961) felt that the loss of a significant relationship was as traumatic psychologically as severe wounds or burns were traumatic physiologically. He argued that grief represented an illness which required a period of time to recover, and he saw mourning as a process of healing through which full health could be restored.

Certainly, bereavement has a powerful impact on the emotions, and troubled emotions can lead to strange and uncharacteristic behaviour which can easily be mistaken for forms of mental illness. Yet labelling grief as an illness is unwarranted for it is an entirely normal reaction to loss, and it is usually quite inappropriate to seek medical assistance for the emotional difficulties that bereaved people face.

Moreover, the medical analogy is doubly unfortunate. The medicalization (the process through which responsibility for coping with natural human events or situations is removed from the individual, and assumed instead by the medical profession) of problems such as bereavement unintentionally attaches to bereaved people the stigma of dependency and helplessness, with solutions arising from medication rather than from within the inner resources of the individual.

Such medicalization too often characterizes attitudes and approaches to the care of ageing people.

Bereavement is, and should be seen not as an illness, but as a normal reaction to loss, albeit one in which normal functioning may, for a time, become impossible. As such, bereavement needs to be treated calmly, with the essentially human 'skills' of sympathy, thoughtfulness, kindness and understanding, all of which are readily available to sensitive, caring people, regardless of training or qualifications.

Indeed, it is the inherent simplicity of the needs of bereaved people that normally requires emphasis, not the specialised professional skills that those needs so often attract.

The scope of loss

Bereavement is caused by significant loss of all kinds. It is important to understand that loss through death is just one of many kinds of loss that people suffer. The grief resulting from death is usually the ultimate, most total, loss, but it is not the only event that initiates catastrophic change; other forms of significant loss, not concerned with death, can be equally distressing. It is important to broaden our understanding of bereavement, particularly in relation to the lives of older people.

Older people are particularly vulnerable to a broad range of loss:

- relationships that fail, or end in separation
- accidental injuries which cause loss of physical or mental abilities
- sudden illnesses which cause temporary or permanent physical or mental loss
- the losses caused by violent, and non-violent crime.

Bereavement, in all these forms, involves readjusting to the emotional consequences of loss in much the same way as people who face loss through death:

- an amputee has to learn to function without a limb
- a blind person must learn to live without sight
- a deaf person must live without hearing
- a person suffering paralysis has to cope with restricted movement.

It is important to realise that the grief arising from a wide variety of physical, emotional and social losses closely resembles the grief associated with loss through death, both for those who suffer the loss, and those close to the bereaved individual.

Loss of physical function and independence

The grief of ageing can begin with the first realisation that the body can no longer accomplish tasks, or does them less efficiently than before. This realisation can arise in many ways, serving as gentle reminders that our bodies are gradually experiencing increased difficulty and tiredness in undertaking tasks once taken for granted.

However, in outlining the deficits that may occur in older age, it is important to stress that such losses are not an inevitable or exclusive consequence of ageing.

Similar decline can occur at relatively early ages, whilst many older people can maintain a satisfactory level of physical performance through into late older age.

The loss of physical function will vary according to individual attitudes, personal relationships, the maintenance of health, and many other emotional and social factors (Scrutton, 1992).

Physical losses

The hair begins to grey, the skin wrinkles, and sporting and recreational activities cannot be pursued with the vigour of youth. Some cherished activities will eventually have to be given up, perhaps through shortness of breath, slower reaction time, or from the tiredness, aches and pains that result.

Loss of vision may give rise to the need for glasses; or the problem may be more severe, perhaps involving visual impairment through glaucoma and cataracts, or through retinal detachment, which may threaten sudden blindness.

Hearing loss may gradually worsen, with many older people reluctant to recognise and accept the fact until it has deteriorated significantly.

These, and other physical losses, may bring with them a growing awareness that life is limited, that we are no longer in our prime, and perhaps can no longer hope to achieve the ambitions and dreams of earlier years.

Diminishing sexual function

The realisation that sexual functioning is declining, perhaps through some diminution of interest, arousal or activity, can cause significant distress. Sexual functioning is closely allied to self-identity, and is also important for the intimacy it can bring to relationships. The capacity to conceive and bear children has passed, an important element in life for many older women for whom childbearing had been a central life-function. Sexual function is an important loss, but one which can often remain unrecognised.

Many of the changes are age-related. Men can experience falling levels of hormonal activity, leading to difficulty in obtaining and maintaining an erection, and lengthening the refractory period. Menopausal changes can lead to gradual changes in ovarian function, reducing levels of female responsiveness, and decreasing vaginal lubrication. The cessation of menstruation may involve losses, representing to some women the loss of youth, femininity and sexual attractiveness.

Yet reduced sexual activity can be brought about as much by the circumstances and inclinations of older people as by their biology. The availability of partners, or the quality of remaining relationships can reduce opportunity, whilst poor health, and social attitudes which are antagonistic to sexual activity in older people, can lead to withdrawal.

The loss of intellectual function

The loss of the ability to think, reason, make decisions, and retain independence in later years is perhaps the most feared loss for older people. Subtle, minimal losses, perhaps indicated by some shortcoming in memory, or some hesitancy or slowness in mental function, may lead to fear about the imminence of much greater losses.

More importantly, intellectual malfunction can be caused by more serious medical conditions, such as some form of cerebral damage, or tumour. The ultimate fear is the progressive destruction of the higher cerebral functions of the brain, through dementia, with its associated anxieties about personal loss of control and the fear of becoming dependent on other people.

Loss through ill-health

With ageing, there is often an accompanying general impairment of health and well-being. Increased dependence on medical care, and increased reliance on medication both threaten an individual's independence and financial security, and can lead to significant loss.

Loss through ill-health can take many different forms, and impact on an individual in a variety of different ways. The long-term or permanent loss of health through illness and disease can lead to:

- the loss of fitness, mobility, and a general feeling of well-being
- the loss of respiratory function through bronchitis or emphysema
- the impairment of mobility through arthritis, or the onset of crippling and degenerative diseases such as multiple sclerosis, leading perhaps to the need for walking apparatus or wheelchairs
- diminished cardiovascular function through heart disease seriously undermining all activity
- the surgical removal of limbs through amputation, the loss of organs, or organ function, having a devastating impact on self-image and self-worth
- the decline of hearing or sight having a serious impact on social functioning
- the progressive loss of mental ability through dementia, often involving the gradual, distressing loss of personality
- strokes, leading to the loss of a wide variety of functions, such as mobility, speech and self-care.

The emotional trauma brought about by such losses can be, and often is, underestimated. They can create a multitude of situations in which an individual becomes aware of a significant loss of personal independence and pride.

The loss of limbs through amputation has been compared with loss through death (Parkes, 1975), and found to take the amputee through the same stages of emotional distress.

The loss of bodily organs, particularly those that have an important impact on personal and sexual identity, such as hysterectomy and mastectomy, can also involve significant losses to a woman's self-image and her feelings of attractiveness and femininity. These factors can be as powerful as a threat to her life. The amputation of male sexual organs, in testicular surgery, although less common, is likely to be associated with similar processes of male grief.

Other severe medical conditions can lead to a dramatic change in body-image. The loss of gastro-intestinal function can be the most embarrassing condition, especially in its more advanced stages involving colostomy (the removal of the stomach) or ileostomy (bypassing the colon), procedures which lead to an altered site for bowel action, and the embarrassment that this can cause.

The emotional trauma that dependency, in all its forms, can bring is not always fully appreciated. Too often even the most caring and thoughtful people respond to

the practical needs rather than the emotional distress,

which often underlay such losses.

It is comparatively easy to see that an individual requires practical assistance; but not always so easy to recognise that this may indicate that the individual also requires support for his/her feelings about becoming dependent on such assistance.

So, merely providing practical assistance, particularly of a personal or intimate nature, can actually undermine the dignity and self-respect of people who hitherto have been fiercely proud of their independence, and defensive of their personal privacy.

Loss through diminishing social involvement

The idea that old age is a time of voluntary withdrawal from social life, and a move towards a self-imposed, but contented isolation, was once a fashionable academic belief (Cumming and Henry, 1961). It remains a common assumption, and for many older people, a self-fulfilling prophecy.

In fact, the reverse process is probably more accurate. It is the way that social life is structured which reduces the opportunities many older people have to remain fully engaged.

The process of ageing often leads to the loss of important social roles, of which the two most significant are the most important roles in life:

- the parental role as children grow up, become independent, and leave home
- the productive work role following retirement.

The personal impact of declining social usefulness and reduced involvement, can be immense:

- a loss of self-value, self-esteem and self-image, with older people feeling increasingly worthless
- reduced income and financial difficulties can lead to an enforced withdrawal from social activity
- a lack of social opportunities to replace friends, through lack of mobility, moving house or area, etc.

When declining health is added to this picture, many older people find that the opportunities of engaging in social life, with the personal fulfilment, direction and purpose this provides, are considerably reduced. This can lead directly to loneliness and isolation, a common feature of the lives of many older people.

Indeed, social withdrawal is often a direct reaction to significant bereavement, creating a vicious circle of loss, leading to loneliness, to social withdrawal and further social losses.

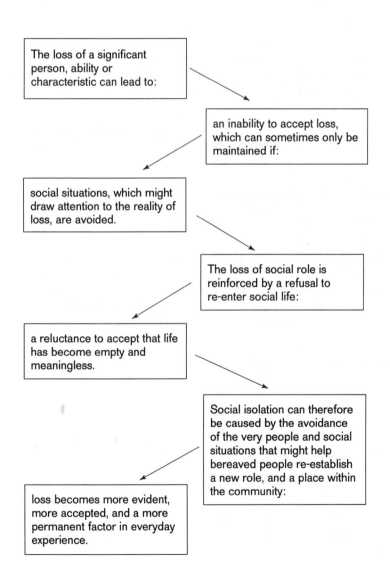

Retirement: the loss of work

Work is usually considered in terms of its functional and financial purposes, but it also has important emotional and social significance. Most retired people will have spent 8 hours per day, 5 days per week, 48 weeks per year in work, for as long as 50 years, yet the impact of retirement is often underestimated particularly for people who have been committed to the challenges of work. Even the recent understanding of the impact of unemployment, discussions about 'the right to work', and the dignity of labour has not been fully applied to retired people, who are capable of work but disqualified on account of their age.

- Work can give meaning to life, a major source of achievement, gratification and self-esteem.
- Work can be a key element of personal identity and social status; the individual is identified as 'teacher', 'foreman', 'doctor', or 'manager'.
- Work may be the basis of personal relationships, a source of focused activity, pleasure and pride.

Even though retirement is seen as inevitable by most people, and desirable by many, retirement for some older people may be unacceptable given their outlook on, and approach to life. More important than this is the loss of a regular daily pattern of behaviour from life. The comfortable familiarity of the place of work, contact with work colleagues, the time spent there, the tasks that filled the day: these all have contributed to the fabric of everyday existence. When they have gone there is often a feeling of emptiness and loss.

One difficulty many couples face after retirement is adjusting to increased time spent together. For some people, this represents the loss of privacy, or private time. Often couples have organized their lives around separate workplaces, different pastimes, habits and friends, and retirement may mean that these have to be reorganised.

Loss of familiar surroundings

Many older people move house, either in response to the need for smaller premises, to accompany the changes of retirement, or because immobility has made their former home uninhabitable. Moving house can result in the loss of familiar surroundings, and detach people from friendship and neighbourhood networks, all of which have been important aspects of social functioning. These former connections can take time to replace, especially when there is no workplace for meeting new people, and financial circumstances and immobility may be constraining influences.

Many older people move to purpose built estates for older people, which may mean that they do not have significant contact with mainstream social life.

Loss of relationships

The process of disengagement assumes that many of the relationships of the older person are willingly relinquished or attenuated, leading to decreased social interaction with people other than with the family.

Yet to describe the loneliness and isolation of older people as a voluntary act in old age is nonsense. Certainly, many former friends may have moved away, died, or no longer call; there are also losses through separation and divorce, or from children moving away from the parental home. Older people often complain bitterly about people who no longer have time for them. They will seek company eagerly, often desperately, becoming reluctant to allow visitors to leave. They miss the companionship that being part of a social group brings.

Older people, particularly those who have become isolated and lonely, feel deeply about their loss of social contact. There is much time spent mourning former friends and relations, whatever the reason for old relationships ending.

Losses through reduced social status

Individuals who feel that they are no longer significant or worthwhile experience a loss in perceived status that can be deeply damaging and emotionally significant:

- retirement removes an important aspect of social status, often allied to reduced financial means, and a reduced sense of purpose and direction in life
- the status attributed to parenting is lost: mankind is one of the few animals not involved in parenting throughout the normal life-span
- social values generally favour the attributes of youth rather than the benefits of older age, such as experience and maturity
- there is loss of independence in later life, which often reaches a climax when older people face losing their homes, and enter institutional care
- the impact of violent physical and sexual assaults affects weaker older people; victims often describe their sense of shock, numbness and disbelief in terms similar to those suffering bereavement
- there is a tendency for older people to withdraw from social interaction, to idealise the past, and denigrate the present.

Such losses are often neglected on the assumption that these are the normal, inevitable consequences of ageing which need to be passively accepted by everyone as they grow older.

Loss through death

The losses arising from death can be immense, and these can be especially significant when a relationship which has endured over many years ends. The loss of a close, loving relationship always creates a void: Somerset Maugham wrote that:

'The tragedy of true love is that one must die before the other.'

The quality of human relationships varies, as will the intensity of grief when they are lost. Some consist of intense, closely knit bonds of close family and friends. Others are less intimate, yet still powerful, based upon the wider family, shared background, and common experience, which have developed into the bonds of close friendship. Then there are complex networks of friends and acquaintances which arise from the community and workplace. Throughout life, this pattern of relationships will provide the individual with the support and encouragement which underlie social functioning.

Older married couples have often spent many years together. Often, the relationship has become comfortable, regular and secure. Indeed, there is usually an over-reliance on the support of the spouse. They know each other well. They have accepted each other's ways, and drifted over the years into mutual dependence. Many older people do not involve themselves socially beyond their spouse and immediate family, thereby depriving themselves of the many potential supports that are available in a wider social context.

For those in later older age, when work has finished, and socialisation has diminished, the marital relationship may even be one of the last close relationships left, the sole remaining source of love and physical affection. The spouse may be the last person who sees value and worth in the individual. Often, a lost partner may have been crucial in providing physical care for the survivor.

When a spouse dies, the survivor may not only suffer an enormous loss of love, but also most of their support system. Life patterns that have become habitual either have to end, or they are continued without purpose. The older the survivor, the less likely they will be to replace the relationship. It can also involve the loss of an important part of 'self', of:

- a lifetime companion, an important attachment figure who has provided love and security
- a source of comfort, support, reliability, relaxation, constancy and security
- a co-manager of the home
- a lover who provided physical, emotional and sexual companionship.

Yet it is not always like this. There can be compensations for the loss of a spouse in older age. Death may have been anticipated and discussed, especially if there was clear warning of death, perhaps through the gradual failure of health, or serious illness. The couple may have talked about what they would do if the other died first, and this can be a helpful preparation for bereavement, although not dulling the intensity of grief that will follow the event.

Other deaths can be equally traumatic. The death of an 'adult' child, or a grandchild, can cause acute grief to older people. However old the 'child', he/she will often remain a child, a part of the parental-self:

- children represent an important lifetime investment in time, love and energy
- they can continue to be the source of love and pleasure
- they can represent the hope for the future, the continuation of family genes.

The death of a child is always untimely, even when they have reached adulthood. The older parent is often deeply disturbed by it, feeling that their own death would have been preferable. Its untimeliness makes adjustment difficult, harder to resolve.

The loss of any important relationship can disrupt many aspects of life for the survivor. The emotional trauma following bereavement can undermine happiness, fulfilment and confidence, the very feelings which support normal social functioning, and give structure and meaning to life. Moreover, grief can arise when the lost relationship has been both unhappy and ambivalent as well as happy.

Even the death of a pet can be a serious loss. Pets can become a primary attachment with isolated, lonely older people, who have perhaps failed to resolve previous losses, for whom their pets have become the chief source of giving and receiving affection, and perhaps a replacement, or link, to the dead person. The death of a pet may lead to a bereavement requiring as much support and understanding as any other loss.

The result of loss through death is that future life can appear to lack purpose, undermining a sense of personal security and identity. Survivors can experience a wide range of uncomfortable emotions, the purpose of which should be clearly understood. Although attention is focused upon the deceased person, and the circumstances surrounding his/her death, the immediate impact of loss, and the principal problem of coping with bereavement, centres around:

the personal losses experienced by survivors.

Dealing with bereaved people is not so much a matter of discussing the loss itself, but enabling survivors to come to terms with their feelings of being:

- alone
- deserted
- vulnerable
- insecure
- empty
- incomplete
- anxious

and the emotional and practical consequences these feelings produce.

The loss of self

The significance of loss for many older people is not restricted to the lost object or person, but extends to the loss of self. Some losses are small, indications of ageing, or partial 'deaths', often taken for granted, but which emphasise that we are mortal, and that death will be the final outcome. Others are more serious – the decline of sexuality, the deterioration of health, or mental ability; each can lead to an increasing preoccupation with personal loss, and eventual death.

This imperceptible relinquishment of life through the gentle fading of body function in ageing people is seen as 'natural death'; but it is no less a loss, and dying in old age is no less significant for the individual.

What will the next deficit be? How will we cope? How will death come? How much life is left to us? All these thoughts lead to varying degrees of fear, the wish to discuss such matters, and to deny such thoughts. There may be an increased concern, an over-interest in personal health; or judgements may be set against the age of parental death, and the survival of brothers and sisters.

The degree of personal concern will vary considerably. For some it may become a consuming interest, whilst others will take it with equanimity. But there will be a growing perception of personal death, and the realisation that whatever happens, we have to meet it alone. Some may wish for a quiet, peaceful, silent, painless death. Some, who feel tired of life, may be prepared for it, and some seem actively to welcome it.

Older people do not need to be ill, or even close to death in order to have such thoughts. Often it is just the recognition that death cannot be too far away. When an individual suffers a major loss, particularly of a close relationship, the sense of personal mortality can be very acute. Such feelings may remain unexpressed, unknown to other people, but they nevertheless constitute loss which can create grieving for the loss of self. And many people do not recognise these feelings, or even that they exist.

Grief

Bereavement is a condition, a situation; it is not, in itself, an emotional feeling. The emotions generated by bereavement are normally described as *grief*. Grieving can be caused by any loss considered significant by the individual. Grief is the normal accompaniment of loss; indeed, the absence of grief following significant loss is usually considered abnormal.

Grief involves a series of powerful emotions which can completely absorb and devitalise the individual. It can produce intense emotional, physical and social pain which at its most insistent can lead to physical weakness, illness, social withdrawal and mental confusion. When life has been shattered bereaved people may experience panic in facing up to the

new realities, feeling that they will never again be able to function normally.

The emotional impact of grief

Bereaved individuals feel acute emotional pain, and many people will
want to add a 'spiritual' dimension to loss.

Grief is a condition that produces a multitude of feelings:

- sorrow
- depression
- bitterness
- guilt
- helplessness
- fear.
- sadness
- anguish
- anger
- regret
- self-pity
- despair
- crying
- frustration
- hopelessness
- longing

Indeed, so great can be the emotional impact of grief that even the
process of living may sometimes often appear too painful for the individual.

The physical impact of grief

Grief can also produce a range of physical symptoms, and a reduced
commitment to self-care:

- exhaustion
- insomnia
- loss of weight.
- tension
- apathy
- restlessness
- loss of appetite

Often health suffers as a consequence, either directly, or indirectly
through recourse to alcohol or drugs, with the individual contracting a
variety of physical and emotional illnesses.

The social impact of grief

The pain of grief can become an impediment to coping with everyday
life. The distress of grief can, at its most extreme, prevent normal social
activities, making life appear worthless, and continued living futile. This
can lead to low self-esteem and self-interest.

No-one, regardless of age, is ever fully prepared for significant loss. A
time of grief can be a particularly bewildering and disturbing period
during which the individual feels depleted, overwhelmed, unable to
cope or function normally.

Many doubt their personal ability to survive, unable to deal with their
suffering. Low self-esteem, and feelings of guilt and resentment can
overwhelm the individual, often for long periods.

Grief: a healing process

Despite the emotional, physical and social trauma of grief, it is important to realise that it is not an unfortunate or unhelpful consequence of bereavement, but an essential part of the process of recovery. This has long been recognised:

- Grief has been seen as a psychological defence against trauma. Freud suggested that mourning is the process by which libido (sexual energy) is withdrawn from a loved object, and that the resulting internal struggle is completed when the ego is eventually freed to continue life.
- Bowlby and Parkes (1970) compared the mourning behaviour of human adults with that of young children and other social animals. When separated from loved ones, the three groups displayed entirely similar behaviour: each cried out, searched restlessly, attacked anything that impeded their search, and sought ways to maintain their memories of the lost person.

Although in the midst of grief it is difficult to be optimistic, it is important for bereaved people and their carers to realise that grief does heal with time, and that they will recover. Moreover, it is important to recognise that the pain of grief is inevitable for anyone leading a full, satisfying life. As Staudacher (1988) says, there is only one way to live without experiencing grief, and that is to exist without loving and being loved. Grief represents our humanity, our need to attach emotionally to other people, and the stress that arises from losing significant people.

Yet grief can be less severe, often unidentifiable, although usually nonetheless painful. Often, individuals faced with significant loss will appear to survive without too many problems. Even so, it should still be recognised that people who appear to be coping well may require support.

The social purpose of mourning and its rituals

Mourning is the period of recuperation from grief following major loss. It is the time during which the individual has to face up to loss, and the apparently intolerable grief that has been aroused. It is, therefore, the beginning of the process of healing and recovery which allows the individual to recommence living again.

The process of mourning is formalised by social expectations. Parkes and Weiss (1983) pointed out that whereas grief is an emotionally-based reaction to loss, producing considerable melancholy, mourning can become a duty to the dead, to other family members, and to wider social expectations. Unless they wish to be considered callous, bereaved people are usually expected to demonstrate grief. It is therefore important to remember that individual reactions to bereavement sometimes have as much to do with how other people believe that they should react as to the way the individual is actually experiencing loss.

Conversely, it is true that the rituals surrounding the mourning process have declined. As Gorer (1965) indicates, there is less expectation for bereaved people to wear black, or to withdraw from social life for extended periods of time. The role and value of the funeral has also declined, and for many people funerals no longer provide an opportunity for 'the unrestrained exhibition of public grief'.

Thus, many bereaved people, whilst conscious of social expectations, are denied some of the traditional opportunities to express their grief, or are uncertain about how they should react. This has led to many bereaved people being treated in ways that are essentially unhelpful, an experience particularly common for older people.

Is bereavement in older age different?

Older age can have a significant effect on how people approach bereavement, and dominant social ideas often suggest that for older people, these effects are usually entirely negative.

Understanding how older people approach the problems of bereavement is important. Throughout life, everyone develops a personal understanding of their world, and an idea of the role they play within it:

> **Everyday objects, and their uses, are identified; personal attachments are made; distinctions are made between friends and enemies; enjoyable and appealing activities are sought, and distinguished from those which are not; as time passes, a distinct, personalised self-identity is formed.**

Everyone interprets their life through these broad understandings, reacting to situations according to their personal perceptions of the world. Each individual becomes involved in activities associated with their particular interests, forms ideas about their personal roles, and the challenges and goals that they want to achieve. Fulfilling these goals (or failing to do so), establishes social status, and the individual gradually develops a sense of self-worth, and personal pride in social performance.

The process of ageing continually changes the nature of these understandings. Each successive life-stage involves a series of gains and losses that can be identified in general terms:

- **As infants:**

| We lose the total protection we once enjoyed as dependent babies. | But we become increasingly able to undertake and achieve actions for ourselves. |

- **Throughout childhood:**
  The imperceptible loss of parental protection continues.

  But we gradually develop skills which increase personal independence and self-esteem.

- **By adolescence:**
  Young people are no longer excused personal failings, purely on the basis of age; they have to assume responsibility for mistakes that, in childhood, might have been forgiven on the basis of inexperience.

  But the adolescent is able to explore many new, exciting enterprises, and experience many new forms of personal relationships previously denied to them.

- **In early adulthood:**
  Each individual develops their optimum physical capabilities and social confidence, and so can seek to attain their maximum prestige and status.

  Yet, adults find themselves in a competitive world where they are expected to assume many duties and responsibilities which restrict their achievement, and personal freedom.

- **In middle age:**
  Greater wisdom and improved social performance can arise from the experiences of life.

  Sometimes the sense of adventure diminishes; some aspects of physical performance begin to decline.

These age-related gains and losses occur gradually over long periods of time. People continually learn to prepare for, adapt to, and accept change, and in doing so, make modifications to their view of the world, and their functioning within it. Even quite major modifications can be made without difficulty, particularly if:

- the changes are gradual
- there has been time to anticipate them
- such change is broadly acceptable to the individual.

Yet if events and circumstances demand modifications that are unwanted, or if those changes invalidate significant parts of our previously assumed role and status, they can be difficult to assimilate.

This is what many older people discover. As people approach the later years of life, there is increasing awareness that some physical abilities are declining, that activities once taken for granted have become more difficult. This represents an experience fundamentally different to any other.

In childhood, we could not perform certain tasks; but then, we never could, and there was the prospect that in time we would be able to do so.

In older age, tasks we have taken for granted can no longer be completed; it is likely we will not regain the ability to do these tasks again.

There are other reasons why older people may not cope well with loss, which arise from generational differences. Many people from older generations were taught to keep their feelings under firm control. They were perhaps told that 'boys do not cry', or that personal problems should be kept to themselves.

This has led to a widespread tendency to underestimate the power of emotional life, and the depth of distress that can be caused by loss. The assumption that people should contain their emotions, show a brave face to the world, and recover as quickly as possible, remains strong. Thus, many older people may tend to display a 'stiff upper lip', to 'snap out' of melancholy and depression, to avoid tears, and have a tendency to believe that grief is unhelpful. Current understanding of grief suggests that this generational response, to the extent that it exists, can run counter to coming to terms with it.

Yet, with ageing there are also gains, even in the process of passing into very old age:

- few older people wish to go through the traumas of youth
- many onerous responsibilities, assumed in adulthood, become less burdensome, or can be relinquished altogether
- the prospect or reality of retirement gives more time to enjoy hobbies and recreations, living on income and pensions earned through a lifetime's toil
- older people possess a body of knowledge and wisdom gained through their life experience
- there are the joys of grandchildren, relieved of the pressures and responsibilities of parenthood
- there are pleasant reflections on life, battles fought, won and lost, and challenges taken up successfully, or in vain.

Older people are often better prepared for loss, and better able to cope with it than younger people. They will have experienced a multitude of different losses and separations which occur throughout life, from birth and weaning, through starting school, going to work, marriage, leaving home, moving house, changing jobs, the traumas of broken relationships, separation and divorce; infertility, stillbirth, miscarriage and abortion; children growing up, and growing away; accidents and natural disasters, the loss of employment, retirement; the onset of serious illness, and hospitalisation, the menopause; the death of parents, relatives, friends and even pets. All these can be an integral part of personal development.

Indeed, older people will have survived the majority of their peer group, and many people younger than themselves. They will have coped with loss in their own ways, some more successfully than others, but the experience will have taught them that they are capable of coping again. It is too easy to underestimate the ability of older people because of our tendency to over-protect, over-care, or to 'infantalize' them.

Loss and death are inevitable parts of human experience. Our ability to cope develops slowly from childhood, through adolescence and into adulthood. In later life, loss may become more constant, more persistent; but the experience remains similar, and our ability to cope unchanged.

Yet dominant perceptions of ageing often disqualify these more optimistic impressions of older age. Instead, the overwhelming view is that older people face a process of decline rather than growth; that there is a period of life when an individual is 'in their prime', after which there exists only decline and degeneration.

This may be an erroneous perception, but it is a powerful one, with an influential impact on reality. Many older people expect to suffer losses, to experience grief as a natural and unavoidable consequence of being old.

These expectations have a powerful way of fulfilling themselves. If we expect old age to be a different, a fundamentally worse experience than any other time in our lives, it can become so.

Such ageist perceptions need to be closely examined by anyone who deals with bereaved older people.

Most approaches to bereavement and grief stress the importance of coming to terms with loss, setting new challenges, and getting on with life. Ageing in a social climate which indicates that there is only an unpalatable future of pain and decline presents additional problems for working with bereaved older people.

Ageism: its impact on bereavement in old age

Losses of all kinds occur throughout our lifetime. Yet loss, rightly or wrongly, is particularly identified with the lives of older people, and considered to be more serious, possibly for a number of reasons:

- older people have less time in which to seek recovery through establishing new relationships and goals; if older people, and their carers, feel that they do not have the time, the energy, or the will to recover, then recovery will be more difficult
- it is assumed that older people have fewer inner resources and strengths to aid recovery
- attachments lost in old age are inevitably of longer standing, and so more important, and less easy to replace
- many older people are reluctant to recognise the importance of feelings, perhaps taught to keep their personal distress to themselves. This is linked to a common tendency to underestimate the power of emotional feelings

- many older people assume that they have 'lived their lives', and should not worry other people with their grief, believing that it is neither helpful or effective to do so.

The accuracy of these perceptions needs to be questioned. Clearly, some of the problems faced by older bereaved people are different owing to the unavoidable circumstances of old age. Yet others arise from different sources:

- the pessimism that surrounds old age within social life
- the restriction and constraints placed on older people, and the way they are allowed to live within society.

Ageist assumptions can make the prospect of loss in old age worse than it needs to be. They pose questions about whether it is important, necessary, or even helpful to bother supporting or caring for older bereaved people.

The dangers of ageism have been discussed in more detail elsewhere (McEwan, 1990); but when negative, ageist attitudes are combined with those surrounding bereavement generally, then bereavement in old age can seem to be, and soon become a devastating experience.

In order to place these ageist factors into their proper context when dealing with older people, there are several factors worthy of recognition:

- loss occurs at EVERY AGE, probably with equal pain and regularity
- there are similarities, as well as differences in the bereavement experience of older people, and the process of recovery is not age-specific
- the serious impact of bereavement on older people is no different to that of any other age, and its significance should not be discounted in any way
- bereaved older people respond to the support and care of those close to them as do people of any age
- many hazards to recovery from bereavement exist within current attitudes and ideas about old age, and these need to be identified and challenged.

Indeed it may be useful to be even more positive than this. In order to develop more constructive approaches to the care of older bereaved people, those who support them need to develop more positive attitudes and approaches to the task. There is evidence that older people are more, rather than less able to adjust to bereavement. McNiell Taylor (1983) stated that older people actually adjusted better than young people to widowhood, in contradiction to popular opinion which continues to believe that they are most seriously affected.

Patronising and disabling older bereaved people

The common assumption that to suffer significant loss after a long and full life is a natural, even timely event, something that should be both expected and accepted, discounts the losses of older people, and inevitably diminishes respect for their feelings.

To use old age to discount the significance of loss, or the genuineness of grief, is patronising and unacceptable.

Conversely, older bereaved people are often treated as the objects of special care and attention, cherished but vulnerable individuals who require protection. All caring responses are based on an implicit assumption that the individual cannot, or should not be allowed to act or make decisions for themselves. Whilst this may be intended as supportive by well-meaning friends, it can be damaging if it is based on the belief that grief is so overwhelming that the individual is unlikely to recover

because of their age.

Such an overreaction to loss in older age underestimates older individuals, and can undermine their capacity to cope. Witnessing the over-caring response of close friends and relatives, they often tacitly accept that they are unable to cope with future life independently.

- **Such a 'caring' response to bereaved older people is disabling and unacceptable.**
- **Bereavement in old age is essentially no different to bereavement at any other time. The experience of loss is no more or less significant at whatever age it occurs.**
- **Therefore it should be taken no more, and no less seriously, and should not elicit a response which is an overreaction, or underreaction to the situation. To do otherwise is disabling or patronising.**

Bereavement and older women

Gender differences also affect the experience of bereavement. Older women were brought up in an era when notions of women's liberation and female emancipation were not significant social ideas. Traditional, male-oriented gender ideas, in which the woman's role was severely restricted, and usually entirely dependent upon their husband, ensures that for many older women the loss of a husband is still a more significant problem than the loss of a wife for a man.

Moreover, the ageing population becomes increasingly a world of women. The greater life-expectancy of women means that two in three people over 75 are women. For some older women, the loss of male company can bring much sadness; for others the prospect of living alone can be frightening. Certainly, they are likely to face four additional problems following bereavement.

Developing a separate, distinct identity

If women have considered themselves as the 'adjuncts' of their husband, without an identity distinct from their former partner, and if this is how they valued themselves, and defined their social role, they can be particularly vulnerable to feelings of worthlessness. Collick (1982) describes how many widows, consciously or unconsciously, feel themselves to be remnants, relics, not people in their own right, with no assured position within the community once bereft of their husband.

The impact on social life

The ability of bereaved women to make new social contacts, to gain introductions to groups, activities and other social events, can be particularly difficult. This is made worse by the tendency for many social events to be specifically geared to couples; many bereaved single women find that they are no longer invited, or feel uncomfortable at functions attended primarily by couples. For many, leisure time is spent with other women, inevitably resulting in a gradual separation from male company. Even female friends can sometimes be unhelpful in this respect, particularly if they perceive that a single woman might be a potential threat.

Often, older women lack assertiveness, a useful asset when attempting to move into new social circles, and many women in this position might benefit from training in this skill.

Reduced income

Many bereaved older women face more severe financial restrictions with the death of their husbands than vice-versa. The traditional division of family roles may also mean that women have been less practised, are less knowledgeable, and therefore less able to organise their financial situations.

Sexual matters

Sexual vulnerability can be another problem older women face following bereavement. Traditional sexual role stereotypes are more influential with most older women, who remain understandably more hesitant to the idea of spending an evening alone in public, or accepting social invitations from men.

2 Social responses to bereavement

Death as social taboo

A characteristic feature of bereavement in modern society is the experience of isolation and loneliness. This arises from a number of key social attitudes and responses that arise from a common uncertainty about what to do, and what to say when facing a bereaved person. This affects the way bereavement is handled, and in turn, gives rise to attitudes which can lead to the avoidance and repression of grief.

It is important to understand the social climate in which bereavement is experienced for two reasons:

- the difficulties this can present to older bereaved people, and how this can prevent them facing up to, understanding, and coming to terms with loss
- so that the supporters of older people can learn to avoid such attitudes, and deal more positively with situations.

Life in Western society no longer fulfils the Hobbesian description of being 'nasty, brutish and short'. In earlier times, people accepted that life was shorter, and had to be prepared to face death. Infant mortality was high, and only a small percentage of people lived into older age. Death was unpredictable and uncontrollable, it took place all around them, and there was an acceptance that death was likely to be violent, and physically painful. People were forced to prepare for death, and there was more awareness of personal mortality.

Expectations now are that life will be both fuller and longer. Modern families no longer experience the regular birth/death traumas of their 19th century Victorian counterparts. Increasing numbers of older people can expect to live into old, and advanced old age.

Yet, this increased life-expectation, rather than developing a more sanguine acceptance of death when it does come, appears to achieve the reverse. Modern responses to death appear to be no better at dealing with its emotional consequences than before:

- social expectations of medical intervention are higher; we no longer anticipate that ill people will die, looking instead to medical cures to prevent death
- death no longer occurs within the home, but in hospitals and other medicalized settings
- contact with the dead body is no longer necessary or desired; it is laid out in 'chapels of rest' rather than the home, where fewer friends, neighbours and relatives choose to view.

These factors have removed death from everyday experience; it is no longer something with which we expect to deal. Although death still surrounds us, most people do not experience it until they encounter it personally, and inescapably.

The result is that we are largely unprepared for death. When it does impinge upon us, we are often aware that it is painful, but the speed and demands of modern life provide little time for more than lingering concern. Then, when it happens too close to our personal lives for it to be avoided, the full impact is felt.

These social reactions to loss place additional burdens on bereaved people who may already be overwhelmed by personal tragedy, making demands upon them which lead to the repression of the mourning process. This can prolong the grieving process, and makes it more difficult for bereaved people to recover fully.

Perhaps the most important single lesson is that death is not a cruel misfortune but a normal feature of life that needs to be anticipated, and accepted.

The denial of death

In contemporary society, the most common response to loss is avoidance and denial. The problem is ignored, in the hope that with time the immediate problems, and the painful emotions, will subside.

Many bereaved people feel that they are avoided, even though bereavement is a time when sympathetic relatives gather in support. Often, conversations are in 'hushed' tones – so as not to 'worry' or 'upset' the bereaved person. Close relatives and friends feel that they are being helpful by not discussing the loss, acting almost as if nothing has occurred that requires open discussion. If the subject of loss is raised, it is often quickly, and embarrassingly changed.

'Giving way to grief is stigmatized as morbid, unhealthy, demoralizing. The proper action of a friend and well-wisher is felt to be distraction of a mourner from his or her grief.' (Gorer, 1965)

This unwillingness to talk to bereaved people can be damaging, excluding those who most need to be included, and denying them an opportunity to express their feelings. Moreover, if the obvious topic of conversation is avoided, it is often difficult to sustain a genuine discussion on anything else; communication becomes strained.

Faced with this general disinclination to discuss loss, many people will repress not only their desire to talk, but also any outward display of emotion. Such restraint can also be damaging to eventual recovery.

The reason often given for denial is to avoid upset, tears and embarrassment to bereaved people. But usually it is not the emotions of the bereaved person that are being spared. Rather more honestly, people will admit that they have difficulty finding the 'right' thing to say.

The more fundamental reason, however, concerns personal discomfort in the presence of distressing emotional pain. Denial arises from a desire to avoid the potential emotional reactions of bereaved people, or doubts about our ability to cope with **our own** emotional responses to the situation. This is, in fact, a quite normal and acceptable reaction. What is wrong, and potentially damaging, is that too often we fail to acknowledge it.

The language of death

The denial of death is reflected in the language that is used concerning bereavement. Our discomfort leads to the avoidance of talking or writing frankly about loss, death and dying. We speak in hushed tones on the basis that it is indelicate, or distasteful to discuss death openly, preferring to talk more optimistically of hopes of reunion and the after-life. A multitude of euphemisms have been created to hide our discomfort about the process of death and dying:

- gone
- passed away
- sleeping
- loss
- deceased
- at rest
- absent
- passed over
- departed
- late
- demise
- expired.

Not dead, but sleeping is a common sentiment inscribed on gravestones – a polite, and apparently harmless description of death and dying.

We assume that bereaved people do not want to hear the words of death, want to avoid them, dread the harshness of their reality. Not speaking of death may reverse what has happened.

Yet good communication at any time is assisted by the use of words which are clear and unambiguous. When dealing with loss it is particularly important that what is said to, and communicated by bereaved people is expressed in terms which are properly understood. Using words which express meaning candidly is always better than empty, guarded or meaningless phrases which, however obliquely, deny the reality of loss.

When language is straightforward, it increases the likelihood that everyone can make sense of what is being said; open, direct language can facilitate the full expression of feelings and pain.

Reassurance

Reassurance can also deny the significance of loss when it consists of bland, meaningless phrases. To reassure is a necessary task in dealing with loss, but not to the exclusion of acknowledging the awful reality that has produced pain and distress.

Bereaved people can be reassured that they are not alone or unsupported; but they cannot be reassured that they have not suffered loss.

Reassurance in the early days of grief are often worthless, mere platitudes and empty words that have little meaning, give no relief, and can be unhelpful:

I know how you feel.	Be brave.
Life has to be lived.	There there.
The pain will end soon.	Cheer up.
Least said, soonest mended.	Give us a smile.
It's going to be all right.	Don't be morbid.
You are doing well.	It's God's will.
You still have your children.	It was meant to be.
You will be fine.	You'll get over it.
You're better off without him.	Don't cry.
Of course you'll find someone.	Crying only upsets you.
Every cloud has a silver lining.	It was meant to happen.

It is usually better to say simply 'I am sorry', or that you do not know what to say. Bland reassurance amidst deep grief cannot be accepted when the immediate pain of loss is too great. Moreover, reassurance can often deny personal emotions, and can be seen to constitute a rejection of the pain they feel:

Reassuring phrase:	**The implied communication:**
• 'There is no need to cry; crying will not help; be brave.'	• I do not want to see you in pain; it upsets me.
• 'Everything will turn out all right in the end.'	• I do not want to face the awful consequences with you.

- 'Pull yourself together; this will not bring him back.'
- 'Have a nice cup of tea.'
- 'Just think of the good times you have had together.'
- 'You will get over it eventually.'

- I am getting annoyed with you, you are upsetting me.
- Let's change the subject.
- I do not want to talk about the unpleasant realities of the present.
- What are you making all this fuss about?

Reassurance can be counter-productive, leading to an awareness that people are either failing to realise the intensity of their grief, or that they do not want to understand. If reassurance is all that is offered, the bereaved person may decide not to express their feelings at all, perhaps in an attempt to avoid further recitation of meaningless, tiresome platitudes. Or they may become angry, even violent towards those who seem content to deny that their distress is genuine.

The fear of death

Death is deeply feared. The result for bereaved people is similar to denial, making it difficult for people to consider loss and death until it becomes necessary, or unavoidable. And then it will prevent full and open discussion of its emotional impact.

The fear of death is concerned with the fear of being alone, the fear of pain, the fear of our emotions, the fear of dependence upon other people. It is shown through avoiding speaking or thinking about it, and denying it when it happens.

The result is often that we avoid coming to terms with it, and in doing so, we fail to live, love, and experience life to the full because we believe in a kind of 'false immortality'. If life consists of an endless supply of 'tomorrows', doing what is necessary to fulfil ourselves 'today' can be left for a 'tomorrow' which ultimately will never arrive. Koestenbaum (1976) suggests several benefits arising from the acknowledgement of death:

- it enables the individual to feel alive, and to enjoy life.
- it makes us aware of the limits of life, and encourages us not to delay doing what we want to do.

In contrast to the secrecy and denial surrounding natural death, the only deaths seen regularly by people are those dramatized on television, usually violent, unnatural, or unexpected deaths, resulting from accidents, murder, or war. As Kübler-Ross (1970) commented:

'In our unconscious mind we can only be killed; it is inconceivable to die of a natural cause, or of old age.'

Perhaps the most illustrative example of society's fear of death is demonstrated by the secretive, back-door removals of bodies from residential establishments for older people. The meaning, purpose and implications of such practice is clear – the desire to remove the dead body without involving or upsetting other residents.

The result is distressing. Often, the first awareness by other residents of death in their midst is an empty chair at the dining table, or lounge. Often there is no explanation for the absence of a former companion, just a gradual realisation that the person is no longer around. Within days, a new resident fills the vacant chair, and death is affirmed.

Tacit within such action is the idea that discussing death, something that many older people want to do, is neither encouraged nor desired. Residents are also aware that their own deaths will eventually be unacknowledged, and treated in the same clandestine manner.

Bereaved individuals, facing denial and fear, learn that people are not willing to listen to their problems at an emotional level. Whilst people may undertake practical tasks on their behalf, the emotional aspects of death seem to be 'forbidden' areas, not to be spoken about openly. The result is that many bereaved people hide their grief so as not to cause upset to people who so clearly do not wish to share it.

At other times, when bereaved people are unable to hide their emotions, it is common for them to be reproached, either being told to 'pull themselves together', or reassured that there is 'no need to be upset'.

Medical attitudes: death as failure

Social denial and the fear of death are emphasised by the activities of one of the most powerful sources of dominant social ideas: the medical profession. Conventional medicine has a problem with death and dying, evidenced by its unrealistic commitment to the maintenance of life at all costs, and the idea that death is diametrically opposed, a contradiction, to its wider mission.

By the 19th century, scientific understanding of medicine and biology led to the idea that both pain and disease could be controlled. Fewer women died in childbirth, disease could be controlled, pain could be relieved, life could become longer and more predictable. Death might also become controllable.

Death came to be seen in terms of causes; the individual was killed by something – a virus, a disease. And if death is caused by someone or something it can be prevented. Medical science has just to understand the causes, and develop strategies – magic bullets – advanced technology – even the replacement of diseased organs – in order to overcome them. The idea that arises is that death can be mastered, even overcome.

The attitude and approach of modern medicine confirm that death represents failure, something to be avoided at any cost. Ill people are taken to hospital, where every effort is made to prevent death. Many patients, who would once have died, are kept alive on life-support machines of increasing complexity, whose purpose is to deny physical death until the last minute – and sometimes well beyond.

The Hippocratic oath has been taken to absurd lengths. Through drugs, complex medical machinery, transplantation, and intensive care units, the extension of physical life has become the paramount consideration. Any failure by medical practitioners to offer the prospect of restoring health seems increasingly to challenge ideas of medical competence. Moreover, these unrealistic hopes and expectations have been passed on to form wider social expectations.

The denial of death, and the social belief in medicine's capacity to overcome it, is taken to its most extreme lengths in the USA, where some companies offer the prospect of renewed life after death. Bodies are frozen, so that they can be returned to life once medical science is able to cure the conditions which caused death.

This medical desire to overcome death implies an over-concern for the physical body, whilst the emotional aspects of preparing people for death are correspondingly neglected. As Parkes and Weiss (1983) stated, there is a real danger that intensive hospital treatment, to the extent that it detracts from the family's ability to care directly for the dying individual, may create additional emotional problems for the family in the period following bereavement.

Perversely, the medical fight against death has produced a reaction which undermines the medical status of older people.

If older people are closer to death, the effort to keep them alive is both more difficult, more expensive, and professionally less attractive. This is fundamental in attitudes towards geriatric medicine which consider it to be:

> 'a second rate speciality, looking after third rate patients, in fourth rate facilities' (BMA, 1986).

In terms of medical priority, older people receive a poor deal from the medical profession. Death cannot be prevented, the end result cannot be modified; working with older people is considered to be 'unproductive' in the face of the futility of old age, and the finality of death.

Other professional groups think similarly. Social work has placed older people, and particularly work concerned with bereavement, low on its list of priorities.

Drugs and medication

In dealing with grief, when the pain of loss is most acute, the use of drugs is a common response. It is a time when many people seek escape from their feelings, and doctors, other professionals, and family members often concur with the prescription of sedatives and tranquillisers. Drugs are commonly seen as a useful way of reducing fear, and offering temporary relief from the unbearable feelings of grief.

Drugs can also provide a message to bereaved people that their feelings are not acceptable. Medication may be an appropriate response in the initial stages of grief, when the individual is in deepest despair, but even then it is usually better avoided. No medication can help an individual cope with grief, or help resolve the emotional turmoil that results. Tranquillising drugs may temporarily numb the senses, and offer the individual some momentary relief from suffering. But such help is purely ameliorative; ultimately medication cannot help resolve grief. It does little more than postpone the time when separation has to be faced, and the new realities of life confronted.

Indeed, the use of drugs may lead to a failure to come to terms with grief, leading to drug dependency rather than an ability to face the new reality. Yet the temptation to use drugs to avoid pain and distress remains strong, and often represents a means by which other people can avoid witnessing the pain of another person's grief, as opposed to seeking a solution to the problems faced by that person.

Insomnia is another normal reaction to significant loss, often involving the persistent recall of the circumstances and consequences of personal loss. Again, whilst such recall can be painful, and sleeping pills are a common means of preventing it, the inability to sleep can be an important aspect of eventual recovery.

Yet medical drugs are not alone in their ability to change reality. Coffee is a drug often used as a palliative to feelings of pain, although its drug effects are not so well known. Following her bereavement, McNeill Taylor (1983) described her addiction to black coffee, based on the surge of adrenaline it caused, and for which she craved. This in turn exacerbated the 'heart flutters' from which she suffered:

'The coffee speeded me up like a junkie. Before long a pot full of acrid black coffee had a permanent place on the side of my stove. It could never be sufficiently black, strong or bitter for me and when other people tasted my favourite brew, they screwed up their faces in disgust.'

Alcohol is another powerful drug often used to blunt feelings of grief. Indeed, McNeill Taylor found that she also resorted to this in order to counteract the effects of coffee; she eventually found that she needed 'a couple of gins' in order to get through the day.

The use of drugs indicates that grief is not being regarded as a natural, healthy, and ultimately a healing process. Bereaved people should be helped to experience and express their pain, rather than to have their feelings suppressed by drugs, whatever their origin.

Where possible, drugs should be avoided, and certainly should not be used as an alternative to listening to the emotional pain that the individual is experiencing.

Religion and religious approaches

Loss will often provoke questions about the meaning and purpose of life and death, why people die, and what follows death. Some bereaved people turn towards religion; others have their beliefs challenged; a few find that former beliefs are seriously flawed.

Religion is a powerful source of dominant social ideology, although it is now much in decline. All human societies, from the earliest times, have evolved rituals and myths in an attempt to give meaning to death. Man has devised many symbolic, primitive, magical and ritualistic ways to cope with the mysterious, fearful and unknown processes that cause death and bereavement, and protecting themselves from it.

For some people, religion remains a major source of solace during bereavement, giving meaning to what has happened, and a framework from which to view and come to terms with death. All religions seem to find ways of dealing with death, and religious belief may provide a means for dealing with loss, as well as a pastoral system of care, both of which can offer genuine comfort and consolation, and give meaning to future life. Religion may also provide a formal acknowledgement of death through some form of final rites.

Clearly, where this is so, religious reassurance can perform a positive role, and can be encouraged. Indeed, the consolation and support given to many older people by religion, with its specific explanation of life, and what is to come after death, can be vitally important.

The ability to share religious and spiritual beliefs with older people following bereavement can be supportive for those who receive solace from religious ideas.

But there should be no attempt to impose belief on bereaved people at such a vulnerable time, as so often happens, for to do so is to take an unfair advantage of bereaved people.

In our secularised society, religious belief is no longer the influence it was, playing little part in people's lives either before or after bereavement. For many people, religious explanations offer little comfort, and to some, seem increasingly irrelevant. For such people it is important that the numerous religious cliches, all genuinely intended to comfort or reassure, are avoided:

- immortality
- everlasting life
- he has gone to a better world
- life has changed, not ended.

Reassurances about the purpose of death, and the idea that the deceased has passed to a 'better world', are satisfactory only to believers in some form of 'life-after-death' in 'heaven'. For non-believers, they cannot replace their strong desire for reunion in **this** world.

Increasing dissatisfaction with religious reassurance is one reason why many former practices, traditions and rituals, which once enabled people to react more appropriately to bereaved people, have withered away. Whereas people would once have looked to the clergy and religious institutions for help, many no longer actively practise religion, and so have no one to whom they can turn.

Moreover, the problems with religious approaches to bereavement are increasingly seen to exist within 'the message' itself. Unlike medicine, religion does not see death as a professional defeat, but as a natural consequence of life. If this were combined with a realistic understanding of the human grief which arises from significant loss, this might be a positive advantage. Unfortunately, religious attitudes have a tendency to discount the significance of 'worldly' death in favour of bland reassurances about the supposed benefits to the deceased who have moved to a better world.

The result is that religious explanations of death, regardless of creed, can appear to discount the personal significance of loss to the survivor. Whatever the message, it is necessary that there should be a clear recognition that loss has occurred, allied to an acceptance that what has happened is significant. In much religious ideology and practice there is a strong tendency to discount the significance of death, and underestimate the problems faced by those who continue to live in this world.

Ethnic and cultural considerations

Loss and bereavement take place in specific social contexts. Different cultures manage bereavement differently, and given that we live in a multi-cultural society, there is a wide variety of social, cultural, ethnic and religious traditions that need to be understood.

In Western society, the process of mourning no longer retains many of the rigid expectations which once defined appropriate dress, behaviour and demeanour, limits of interaction, and the period of time considered appropriate for the public expression of grief. It now relies upon less defined, more individualistic responses. Gorer (1965) has suggested that present day difficulties in coping with bereaved people are largely due to this lack of established ritual, and structured patterns of mourning.

In contrast, many non-Western communities have retained a more fertile set of traditions, consisting of clear moral codes, widely accepted belief systems, honoured customs and rituals, allied to strong expectations of community support. The meaning of death is defined, and the nature of grief and mourning are specified, all designed to help bereaved people through loss and the process of recovery.

Supporting bereaved people from different cultural backgrounds needs to involve an acceptance of the individual's view of the world, and this has led to differences of opinion about the value and possibility of cross-cultural support:

- some people believe that sensitive support, based on the counselling skills of listening, empathy and positive regard can be sufficient to enable cross-cultural support, even without a detailed knowledge of specific belief structures, or our own personal racism
- others believe that our own experience of race and culture within a racist society makes it difficult for effective cross-cultural support to take place
- another view suggests that it is possible to gain a sufficient understanding of different racial or cultural differences to facilitate effective support, but that this knowledge is essential, and should include a knowledge of how discrimination and racism within contemporary society can affect people from minority cultural backgrounds.

Many people believe that culturally determined attitudes towards loss and bereavement, the ceremonies and rituals of traditional cultures, serve the emotional needs of bereaved people well, often providing direct and acceptable channels for the expression of sadness and anger, and adequate guidelines for the duration and conclusion of mourning.

Yet we should not become sentimental about traditional values. For many people they can be rigid and stultifying, and are seen as increasingly irrelevant. Any tradition or belief is valuable to an individual in direct relation to its acceptance, and certainly traditional values cannot be re-established on a wave of sentimentality.

Moreover, assumptions about cultural and religious beliefs based on racial stereotypes can be unhelpful. It is always best to check with individuals, regardless of their background, about personal beliefs and expectations throughout each period of mourning.

Yet when people have strong beliefs and acceptance of cultural norms, it is important that their normative values, customs, practices and beliefs are understood in order to respond sensitively to their wishes and needs.

This can be particularly important with older bereaved people, many of whom will be first generation immigrants who may have hoped to return to their 'roots' prior to their old age, and who may retain greater commitment to traditional values than younger family members, who may have modified cultural values, and become more 'Westernised' in outlook. Such generational gaps may become increasingly apparent.

Sometimes, older members of minority ethnic communities find that they have only small networks of support for traditional rituals, and some may find it difficult to cope with the breakdown of traditional values and respect, and become prone to prolonged mourning and personal breakdown.

The complexity and variety of belief cannot be tackled here; where support comes from relatives and close friends, aware of cultural background and belief, this will be less important. Yet it is important to stress that as society has become more complex, mobile and multi-racial, it has also become highly individualistic, with belief structures losing their influence over families and communities.

There remains much that is common to different cultural groups however. Most provide some outlet for:

- the public expression of emotion, whether sadness, anger or aggression
- the recognition that bereaved people are in a state of shock and disorientation, and require support, care, feeding, and comfort
- some understanding, and often fear that the spirit of the deceased remains behind in some form after physical death
- provision for the correct or expected method of disposal of the body
- a final post-burial ceremony which confirms the finality of loss, and indicates to bereaved people that it is time for recovery and reintegration into social life.

Moreover, the process through which bereavement passes (Chapter 5) does not vary significantly between different cultures. The emotional responses felt and expressed by people from different cultural backgrounds remain similar.

Despite this, it is important to recognise that complex issues of culture and race may arise when a carer and a bereaved person come from different cultural and racial backgrounds. This does not have to be through directly prejudicial or racist attitudes. Relationships can be hindered, even destroyed, by an inadequate knowledge of cultural differences, subtle differences in attitude and approach, an inappropriate use of language, non-verbal behaviour, and inaccurate assumptions.

3 Initial responses to bereavement

Time, it is often said, is a great healer. To the extent that this statement is a truism, it offers little comfort to those in the early stages of grief; indeed, it can seem to belittle and discount the importance of their current distress, and reference to it should be avoided. Yet recovery from bereavement does rely heavily on the passage of time, and the more creatively this time is used the more complete recovery will eventually be.

Who should respond to bereavement?

The more significant the loss, the more difficult it becomes for the bereaved person to cope without help and assistance; as William Shakespeare intimated:

'Everyone can cure a grief but he who has it.'

When a person has suffered significant loss the experience can vary in intensity between being slightly unnerving, to causing acute social and emotional distress, leading to the possibility of longer-term debilitation. The potential impact of loss has led to an assumption that professional intervention should be provided to deal with intense grief, and that untrained people have little to offer.

So who should provide assistance to bereaved people? Should we help? Are we capable of doing anything helpful? What can we do about our own doubts and feelings? Would it not be better to call on a professional?

Many such understandable apprehensions exist. Indeed, there has been a tendency throughout the 20th century for problems that would once have been settled within the family or the immediate community to become matters dealt with by professional carers. One example has been the tendency to 'medicalize' the process of death and bereavement (a process by which medical personnel have taken increasing responsibility for caring for sick, dying and bereaved people on the assumption that this was supportive to the family, giving reassurance and relief from stress).

Alongside medicalization has been increasing emphasis on individual work, as opposed to work with families and friendship groups. Similarly, the value of working within such supportive groups is now being rediscovered.

Both medicalization and individualisation are being re-examined. Together they have deprived the family of many opportunities to care for dying and bereaved relatives, undervaluing its potential caring role, and the benefits the family's involvement can offer all parties in the mourning process.

The trend is increasingly to recognise that grief is a social process, best handled within social settings within which people can support and reinforce each other in loss. Bereavement seldom affects the life of just one individual; usually entire families and networks are affected, each person to varying degrees, and each in turn affected by the powerful emotions experienced by other members of the social group.

Most evidence suggests that families that have open and effective communication can share, and facilitate the expression of grief, and can be helpful in assisting recovery. Most older people retain a network of family and friends who are able to play a supportive role. Moreover, unlike professional intervention, the support of close friends and family is not usually time-limited, but available on an on-going, life-time basis.

When families are able and willing to offer a reasonable standard of physical care, and this can be provided with sufficient emotional and social support, family members usually prefer to cope themselves, despite the difficulties and inconvenience this can involve. The more sensitive family members are more likely to become part of the helping process, and ultimately more likely to offer bereaved people effective support and improved care which has several advantages:

- the individual can be cared for by those people who have been most important in their life
- family members and friends are provided with an opportunity to make restitution for any past failures, misunderstandings, or inadequacies
- dying and bereaved people usually feel happier, less lonely and more supported amongst people they know, and within familiar surroundings
- the intense emotions of bereavement can often be assuaged when family members are able to care for dying and bereaved relatives
- the value of mutual grieving, the simultaneous process of helping and being helped, can be utilised
- it recognises that loss is a normal and inevitable part of family life.

Whilst there are several people and organisations which can be called upon to provide help for bereaved older people, the type, duration and quality of the help offered varies considerably. A variety of voluntary and professional agencies, ranging from church clergy, the Red Cross, St John's, St Andrew's, the WRVS, various local and national charities, the Council for Voluntary Service, Age Concern, Social Service Departments, including social workers, home help staff, and care staff at elderly people's homes, doctors, district nurses, health visitors, occupational therapists, nurses, alternative medical practitioners, even local counsellors, might be available.

CRUSE (bereavement care) requires a special mention as a voluntary organisation, which trains and offers well-trained counsellors who specialise in working with grief. The organisation is now established in most towns and cities, and both bereaved people and carers can call upon their services.

Yet the reality of the current political climate, particularly when allied with the low social priority and status of older people, means that there are severe limits to the availability of such help. The provision of professional community support for bereaved people has declined in recent years, and in any case, it should be recognised that few professional staff are specifically trained in grief work with older people. There is also evidence from research evaluating professional help suggesting that the quality of communication and support can be poor, and that it does not produce significantly better outcomes than 'informal' networks of care.

Reliance on professional support can be part of the denial and fear of death. Often, the failure to offer 'informal' support arises from embarrassment or awkwardness. Many people feel that they have nothing to offer, preferring instead to call on others, and in doing so, relinquish personal responsibility. When faced with another person's grief, even close friends can recoil from active involvement, preferring to avoid facing their pain, perhaps relying upon the less personal contact of cordial letters, cards, and flowers.

It is easy to condemn such impersonal responses, but important to understand that they often arise as much from uncertainty and unfamiliarity with grief than from any spiteful intent.

There has also been a decline in extended family networks, and close neighbourhood ties which once provided support systems for people suffering loss. Many older people now live in isolated units, either individually or in small groups where there are few people to share problems, or to create adequate support systems.

The result is that more older people find themselves unsupported, and fewer people are available to offer support.

If the task is to be undertaken, it often has to be done by those who are available, and those who care sufficiently for the individual, quite regardless of their training and experience. Fortunately, the help people require does not need to be trained, professional support. Bereavement is a social process. Many people, including:

- family members
- close friends
- neighbours
- former colleagues
- people who have experienced similar loss

have contact with bereaved people, and may be called upon, or find themselves in a situation, where they can offer invaluable comfort and consolation.

Older bereaved people are often supported informally by people willing to offer uncomplicated assistance which arises from their sensitivity, patience, and genuine concern for the individual. What they offer does not emanate from special training or qualification, but can be supportive in many ways:

- simple friendship
- someone to talk to
- someone to hold, and to cry with
- someone to provide a reassuring presence
- someone to undertake helpful practical tasks.

Many people find such help to be more acceptable than professional intervention. Smith (1982) argued that humility and respect are more valued qualities than 'flashy therapeutic skills', and that the role of the familiar comforter is as relevant as ever. Schiff (1977), writing about the death of her child, argued that bereaved people can often gain more comfort, understanding, and hope from people who have suffered similar losses. Many caring people, who would have much to offer bereaved older people, fail to do so for these reasons, and fail to appreciate the value of gentle words of comfort, the confirmation of mutual affection, and simple friendship.

However, many people do not feel they have any choice: a close friend or relative is suffering, and they must help if they can. Often, there is no-one else able or willing to do so.

Personal commitment: the implications of offering support

'The loss of a loved person is one of the most intensely painful experiences any human being can suffer, and not only is it painful to experience, but also painful to witness, if only because we're so impotent to help.' (Bowlby, 1980)

There are many problems involved in supporting bereaved people. Often, help is offered too readily, without careful consideration of personal implications. The task is usually emotionally taxing, with even intimate friends and relatives becoming exhausted by trying to help people through grief. It can even challenge close friendships unless the problems and difficulties are faced and understood.

To support bereaved people, the individual must recognise the difficulties of the task, and the personal difficulties that can arise. There are four main considerations:

- Is there sufficient personal commitment to the bereaved person to facilitate the required level of support for the duration of grieving?
- Do we have sufficient time, personal strength and skill to cope with profound grief?
- Can we cope with the personal stress caused by close proximity to the pain of bereaved people?
- Do we have adequate support systems to enable us to offer support?

It is extremely painful to witness intense grief. Before making a commitment, individuals must decide whether they can tolerate the stress of being close to the pain, suffering, and helplessness of the bereaved person. It is certainly easier to withdraw, or to seek to discourage its expression by telling them to 'pull themselves together', to 'stop crying', or in some other way to deny their pain, or hurry them through the mourning process.

If there is any reluctance to cope with such feelings, the individual might not be able to encourage the full, open disclosure of emotions that is usually necessary for recovery. Caring successfully for bereaved people means allowing them the opportunity to grieve fully; to deny this serves only to prolong and intensify the mourning process. Anyone intending to work with bereaved people has to be prepared to face the personal emotions that can arise from close proximity to grief. This can bring the carer closer to the fragile nature of life and death, which inevitably heightens awareness of the delicate nature of personal mortality.

For this reason, self-knowledge is helpful. Carers should have come to terms with their own fears and feelings about loss in their own lives, and their attitude towards death, for it is important that personal feelings do not interfere in the helping process. This can also help determine personal limitations in terms of how helpful we can be.

Personal stress can be particularly acute when the carers are affected by the same loss. Close relatives are sometimes not the most appropriate people to offer support when they are grieving themselves. Conversely, their commitment is often greatest, and to share the process of grieving with others can often be mutually supportive.

Support for supporters

No professional person would undertake grief counselling without supervision. Similarly, relatives and friends should expect to receive support too. The helplessness often experienced by older bereaved people can be frightening, particular where there are concerns that they may become dependent on us on a long-term basis.

Moreover, the reaction of bereaved people can often involve hostility toward those who offer help, and this can leave carers shocked, disappointed, and alienated. The local GP or social services department should be able to provide suitable support, or guide the individual to where it can be provided, perhaps through local support groups for carers, counselling groups, or groups which focus on the care of older people.

No person undertaking work with bereaved people should feel obliged to do so without adequate support and assistance. Ask: and if the response is not adequate, ask again. If necessary, keep asking, and if necessary, complain; do so until you receive support which you feel is acceptable.

The benefit and purpose of having support is twofold:

- **Personal:**
  It should enable carers to discuss personal feelings which arise from close proximity to grief. Deep feelings of loneliness, emptiness, fear, anger, guilt, and even suicidal despair, can be daunting, and if carers are to remain responsive to people's grief they need an outlet to express their feelings in order to survive them, restore themselves, and continue to offer support.
- **Practical:**
  Carers can be uncertain about what to do, or how to respond to situations. It is helpful to be able to discuss such doubts with someone who is able to offer practical guidance and advice. Support can offer carers an opportunity to develop the skills and techniques which will assist their support, alongside a deeper understanding of the process through which bereaved people are passing.

Just being there: a reassuring presence

It is important to accept that it is quite normal to feel ill-at-ease, to worry about correct behaviour, to be lost for words, or to want to say the right things. The stressful emotions surrounding work with older bereaved people means that it is not easy to know what to say, when to say it; when to stay and help, and when to leave; when to console, and when to provoke.

In fact, it is the most natural, simplest responses that are most important. Tatelbaum (1981) offers sensible advice; try at all times to be sensitive to the needs of bereaved person, and use the 'rule of thumb' test:

What you would like people to do for you if you were in a similar position?

When in doubt, it is acceptable to ask directly: if they want to be quiet, then be quiet; if they want to talk, then talk; whatever happens, do not rush to fill silences.

The most valuable gift relatives or friends can give in the early stages of bereavement is their companionship and time, perhaps sharing personal memories and anecdotes. Most people require support to enable them to face the mourning process. The experience of loss can lead to a depletion in energy, and the simple presence of other people is often vital to prevent them having to experience their fear and anguish alone. Loneliness can serve to accentuate personal despair, and highlight feelings of emptiness and hopelessness.

The acknowledgement that we understand that their loss is meaningful to them and us, something that can be said simply and directly, can be important, as can all caring and supportive responses. They help bereaved people feel that they are not a burden, that their feelings are being recognised, accepted and understood, and that our attention to their needs is freely given.

The value of inactivity

It is not activity that gives comfort, but being receptive to, and understanding of the individual's pain and distress. It is often sufficient to be present, in the same room, sitting close, without doing anything, just offering a listening ear, and demonstrating personal concern.

An inactive presence can provide bereaved people with support and reassurance, an awareness that someone is, and will continue to be available for them. The value of this is inestimable: it is certainly more important than any professional advice or expertise.

Yet whilst it is unnecessary to be busy with practical tasks, the urge to be active can be powerful, often based on the idea that:

life must go on.

This is especially so when the bereaved person may feel that life for them has ceased, or when they may want it to do so. Thus, it is often helpful to curb the desire to 'do something' which is best left undone, or to 'say something' which is best left unsaid.

Silence

There exists a powerful, but largely erroneous belief that there is a 'right' way to act, and that there are 'correct' words to use. Offering a caring, supportive presence, being a good listener, and perhaps saying 'I'm sorry', are usually more important than any particular form of words.

Silence is also acceptable. It can represent a comfortable, even intimate, sharing of time, a chance for bereaved people to experience their feelings, without being challenged or pressured. Silence does not have to be 'empty', and can indicate an acceptance and understanding that there is nothing that can usefully be said, or that people must struggle to find their own words, in their own time, to express their feelings.

Patience is necessary in the initial stages of grief; discomfort and embarrassment should not lead to pressure to start a conversation, or to embark on meaningless chatter, or to resort to worthless platitudes. We should be prepared to sit silently if this is what the individual requires.

Staying or leaving

For recently bereaved people, company is often necessary, and carers should be available, for when support is withdrawn suddenly, or without warning, it can be interpreted by bereaved people as another loss.

It can take many weeks to come to terms with loss, and bereaved people may require consistent support throughout this time. In the early days it may be necessary for a group of friends and relatives to form a 'rota' to ensure that the bereaved person is supported, but to enable other people to attend to their other responsibilities.

However, whilst company is essential for most people, some individuals may genuinely want to spend time alone. We need therefore to be sensitive about how long we stay. It is certainly possible to stay too long, particularly if the bereaved person does not like to ask us to leave, or does not know how to do so.

Physical contact

Physical contact can provide bereaved people with considerable reassurance. Sitting close, touching, holding hands, an embrace, passing a tissue, crying together, are all simple gestures which demonstrate care and sympathy, and often do so better than any words.

For many bereaved people, and their carers, physical contact may be a natural response. Simple touch can convey the very humanity bereaved people may feel they have lost. It can demonstrate that another person is sensitive to their pain.

Yet for others, the tenderness associated with physical contact can be frightening, especially for older people brought up in a less tactile age.

There may be hesitancy or embarrassment arising from the close association between touch and intimacy. The fear of rejection can arise if touch might contravene some personal boundary.

Physical contact is important, but it is not crucial; it will depend upon the relationship, but in all situations, it is necessary to respect the wishes of the individual. It may come more easily to women than men, as physical contact is so often associated with weakness, or suggestive of sexuality.

Listening

When bereaved people wish to express their feelings, the simple act of listening and acknowledging their sorrow and pain is often sufficient. Often we will feel unable to offer a meaningful reply, and this is acceptable. Perhaps we just need to share with them our helplessness; we would like to help relieve their pain – but there is little or nothing that we can do to achieve this.

The feelings of the bereaved person should be the central focus of attention. Often bereaved people will want to repeat endlessly the things uppermost in their mind. The role of the carer is to help them express themselves. Sometimes, in the early stages of grief, carers can only listen to bereaved people reliving the events leading to loss, reviewing the nature and significance of their loss, and expressing doubts and worries about the future.

Through listening and demonstrating genuine concern, even if this is shown by a nod of the head, or a consoling touch, the carer can help the individual maintain some sense of personal value and worth through a difficult time.

Yet there are many distractions to listening which need to be limited as much as possible:

- telephones ring
- well-wishers visit
- televisions and radios distract
- young children and animals divert attention.

Listening can be assisted by an open and relaxed posture, avoiding crossed arms and legs, a reassuring facial expression and sympathetic eye contact.

Our attitude is also important. We need to display genuine concern, acceptance, and empathetic understanding, all matters dealt with in the next chapter when the art of listening is considered in more detail. We also need to conceal personal fears and anxieties which can arise when working with bereaved people.

Comfort and consolation

The appearance and behaviour of bereaved people will usually evoke caring responses.

The body is crouched, the head is lowered, shoulders are hunched, the face is anguished, and there is distress, tearfulness and weeping.

Comfort and consolation are necessary at acute times of loss; indeed the most basic human responses to personal grief and suffering is to hold, touch, to offer sympathy. But in doing so, it is important that carers do not collude with denial, or other defences which can hinder eventual recovery.

It is also important to recognise that no support offered can prevent the feelings associated with loss. If there is longing for the deceased, bereaved people will want only reunion. The only way that their pain can be relieved is for them to recover what they have lost, something that bereaved people often secretly desire. No-one can or should offer this.

All that can be done is to offer consolation for the pain that separation has brought them.

Our support is inevitably limited. It enables the bereaved person to feel that someone cares, and wants to support them through their suffering. Indeed, sharing grief with another person can be helpful, but our failure to give them what they want can lead to our efforts to console being rejected. If we cannot make things right, we become only a further, hateful reminder of their loss. Relationships with other people, including our relationship, however close and meaningful it may have been, may not be wanted, or may fade into insignificance in comparison to their longing for reunion.

Carers can feel spurned and unwanted. The role of the carer is to accept this as the initial price they have to pay to offer meaningful support. The feelings of the bereaved person are central, and we have to allow them full and free expression, however hurtful this may be.

There is no easier way, certainly not by deluding people with ultimately unhelpful ideas about reunion. No-one can offer consolation if all people require is the return of what they have lost. Whatever comfort and consolation can be offered, it should not contradict reality.

Facilitating emotional release requires assisting bereaved people to recognise and express their feelings, to recognise the new reality, to come to terms with it, and what it means to their future life.

Practical tasks

The most obvious response to the question of 'what to do', and one which most people find the easiest to undertake, is to tackle the various practical tasks, of which there are many that may need to be done:

- contacting undertakers, making funeral arrangements
- notifying friends and relatives
- preparing and eating meals
- answering the phone
- shopping, running errands
- tidying the house, cleaning dishes
- listing those who wrote, bought gifts, sent flowers
- replying to letters, and notes of sympathy
- acting as a spokesperson, or intermediary
- protecting people from 'unwelcome' visitors.

There may be other specific tasks to undertake. For example, bereaved people may wish to avoid certain rooms or places associated with the deceased, or they may feel unable to deal with the personal effects, the clothes, belongings and equipment of the deceased.

Sensitivity to the needs and feelings of the bereaved person is required in offering practical support. Blindly getting involved in essential tasks may appear straightforward, particularly if bereaved people are in no position to ask for help, or do it themselves. But many older people may want matters left as they are; they may resent, or be irritated by any form of practical assistance which may be seen as an intrusion. Or the task might be done incorrectly, at the wrong time, or offend in some other way.

Even well-intentioned help can often be misunderstood, and can in some circumstances lead to conflict. Therefore:

- decide what needs to be done immediately and what can wait until the individual can make personal arrangements
- prioritise the tasks that need to be undertaken pro-actively, rather than waiting to be asked.

There is also a danger, implicit in all 'caring' responses, of disabling the individual. By focusing on the practical, physical needs of the older individual, and making them feel that they are no longer capable of doing things for themselves, we only create dependence on the support of other people. Most older people do not want to be dependent, and the association between age and dependency can make them more sensitive about doing things for themselves.

So whilst undertaking some practical tasks may be important, it is always necessary to help bereaved people regain their own self-confidence and involvement by assisting them to take responsibility for what needs to be done, albeit with relevant advice and support.

Decision making

During the initial mourning period, decisions may need to be made. Bereaved people often have little interest in deciding anything, particularly when the deceased was the major decision-maker within a relationship. Moreover, decisions made when stressed, depressed or apathetic do not usually produce the wisest long-term outcomes. It is often best to wait, if this is at all possible.

Major decisions, such as moving house, selling possessions, or removing belongings that may serve as painful reminders of the deceased, should be left. Premature action on such matters often proves to be mistaken. When mourning is complete, quite different decisions may have been taken. For example, the bereaved individual may have personal possessions that, in the midst of grief, are too painful to see, but which later can bring back cherished memories.

Patience and acceptance

Carers need to accept the validity of the attitudes, feelings, concerns and actions of the bereaved person. There should be no attempt to compare, evaluate or judge the behaviour of bereaved people for this serves no useful purpose. Acceptance, without being patronising or causing provocation, is the best response in the early stages of grief.

The carer may need to be patient with violent mood changes. Spending time with bereaved people can be uncomfortable, especially during the early stages of grief when there may be a strong desire for reunification with the deceased. They may resent or ignore your presence, and carers may even be subject to blame, anger, and rejection – all normal aspects of the grieving process. It is often difficult to accept the behaviour of bereaved people, but such behaviour should not be taken personally.

Gratitude

The personal rewards arising from supporting bereaved people can be minimal. There should be no expectation, no matter how much time and energy are spent, that the reward will be gratitude. This may come eventually; but certainly cannot be counted upon during the initial stages of bereavement. Indeed, supporting grieving people can be difficult:

'(This) stems from the awareness of both parties that neither can give the other what he wants. The helper cannot bring back the person who's dead, and the bereaved person cannot gratify the helper by seeming helped.' (Parkes, 1972)

It may also appear that our efforts produce little significant result, and that there are few rewards for what can seem to be a painful and time-consuming endeavour. Indeed, if the task ever seems to become easier, or less complicated, the carer is probably beginning to deny, or block some of the reality of the bereaved person's grief.

Special times

The various rituals and ceremonies surrounding bereavement can be both helpful and unhelpful. Perhaps one function of support is to make such occasions as helpful as possible during the process of mourning.

Viewing the body

Most evidence suggests that viewing the body is an important part of the adjustment process. It can confirm the final reality of death, helping individuals to begin the process of working through their grief. It provides:

- an opportunity to see and become familiar with the reality of death
- an opportunity to see, touch and hold the dead person, and time for last farewells
- a private time together for reminiscence, regret, and sadness.

Many people claim that to witness the peaceful expression on the face of the deceased can be helpful in coming to terms with death.

So although viewing the deceased's body can be traumatic, it does allow bereaved people to take the first step from disbelief to belief, particularly when death was sudden or unexpected, or when it took place in their absence. However, there is often reluctance to view the body. Some people insist that they want to remember the dead 'as they were'; others find the idea abhorrent, and recall the event later with considerable distress. This can be particularly painful when an individual is asked to identify the body following a death involving gross physical injury.

There is also a reluctance by some relatives to allow older people to view the body of a loved one, in order to protect them from the pain that this might involve. There may also be medical, legal or bureaucratic restraints which may limit the duration of viewing, or insist on viewing through a screen, or prevent touching or holding the body.

People who, for whatever reasons, are denied contact with the body, perhaps when it cannot be found or is badly mutilated, can find it more difficult to accept the reality of the death, and this may delay the eventual recovery of bereaved people.

Some older people, who have been prevented from viewing the body, or attending the funeral, perhaps because it was considered too distressing for them, feel considerable resentment about their exclusion. It often leaves them confused about what has occurred, and isolated from the new reality of life.

Where there is resistance to viewing the body, from whatever quarter, decisions have to be made about how this can be overcome. If it is part of the denial of death, and might slow the recovery process, some gentle encouragement may be sufficient to change a person's viewpoint. Even after the event, this can be rectified by visits to the grave to enable the individual to grasp the reality of what has happened.

The funeral

The role of funerals has attracted considerable criticism in recent years. They have tended to become highly formalised, impersonal events, their value further restricted as they usually take place very soon after the event when the immediate family and close friends may still be too dazed or numb to understand the full significance. This can reduce the positive impact funerals might otherwise have.

The commercialisation of death has been particularly unhelpful. Mitford (1963) has outlined the bizarre history of American funerals where they have become big business. Morticians, using sophisticated sales techniques, have transformed funerals from the simplicity of former times, where the body was placed in a plain pine box, and the 'laying out' of the deceased was done by friends and family, who also bore the coffin to the grave, to a position where they have become status symbols of staggering expense.

Yet funerals can still be a positive feature in the process of recovery from grief, symbolising many things to different people, and fulfilling many functions for the living:

- The funeral can help people recognise that loss has occurred, representing the passage of the body from this world to another, separating the dead person from the living. It can provide the first appreciation of the significance of what has occurred.
- The funeral provides an outlet for the expression of public grief, and the communication of sympathy and concern. This can demonstrate that the individual is not alone in his or her loss, and the funeral can provide an opportunity for shared grief.
- The funeral is a farewell, a public opportunity for friends and relatives to say goodbye together. It can be a positive celebration rather than a negative farewell which focuses on distress and pain, an expression of gratitude for the deceased, confirming that he/she has made a mark on the lives of other people which will ensure that they are remembered and valued.
- A funeral can indicate that death is part of the essential pattern of life,

signifying that the deceased person will continue to be significant to both the family and the wider community.

- A funeral can bring together widely scattered social networks, and be a social occasion during which family and friends can provide mutual support, spend time together, revive or renew family bonds and former relationships, and offer support to those most affected.
- A funeral can offer an opportunity for people to reminisce about the events and circumstances of the deceased's life, their thoughts and feelings about the deceased, and place his/her life into some perspective. In particular, bereaved people can be encouraged to speak about the impact of their loss on future life, thereby starting the essential process of discussion and reflection.
- A funeral can begin the process of separation, a time when bereaved people should begin redirecting their lives on the understanding that this will be spent without the deceased.

The period after a funeral can be difficult. The sudden flurry of social activity, the renewal of former contacts, can quickly be followed by a feeling of intense loneliness when they have left. For the main carers, on-going companionship and continuing assistance beyond the funeral are important.

Symbols and anniversaries

Following loss, there will be many reminders of the past. Symbols and anniversaries associated with the deceased will be abundant, particularly at the end of a long-standing relationship:

- a favourite song played on the radio
- a favourite television programme
- household memorabilia
- personal belongings
- favourite flowers
- special times of the day associated with the deceased
- birthdays
- wedding anniversaries
- the anniversary of the bereavement
- the first Christmas or Easter alone.

There are many other notable times that can lead to thoughts and feelings about the past which may bring fresh grief and mourning when an individual may require extra support. This can be worse when they occur shortly after the bereavement, but they can arise even after the main grieving process seems successfully to have passed. Such reminders of loss can generate feelings of renewed loneliness, and can lead to intense feelings of panic, distress and many other physical symptoms.

Yet despite their importance, the commemorations of these and other anniversaries are often either forgotten or overlooked by friends, sometimes in error, and sometimes intentionally so as not to cause further distress. Carers should be encouraged to note special dates so that arrangements to support the individual can be made. In this way potential problems can be anticipated. Even so, there are still many questions that need to be considered:

- Which are the important anniversaries?
- How is it best to respond to them?
- What is the best way to ensure that the memory of the deceased is maintained?

When these have been determined, a card, a note, or a visit to confirm that the deceased is still remembered can be helpful in reassuring bereaved people that the deceased person lives on within the memory of other people.

In residential units, dealing with death can be assisted by regularly remembering former residents on the anniversary of their deaths, either informally, or through prayers and services to their memory. This would reassure living residents that they, too, will be remembered after they die.

Sleep, rest and dreams

In times of distress, rest and sleep are important aids to restoring physical and mental energy, and the maintenance of health and strength. Often, however, the grieving mind is too busy, too hurt to allow it peace. Then, lack of rest can weaken both body and mind, undermining the individual's ability to cope.

Many older people become worried if they do not sleep properly. Insomnia takes many forms, and arises from many factors. It may result from an over-active mind, or a fear of falling asleep, especially significant after someone has died in their sleep. Fitful sleep is another problem, with frequent waking after short periods of sleep, often followed by an inability to sleep further. Others find that even after long periods of sleep they do not feel fully rested on awakening.

Yet the value of rest and sleep has to be balanced against the need for bereaved people to experience personal thoughts about their loss. Troubled and painful thoughts are part of the process of coming to terms with what has happened. An active mind, going over loss at the expense of sleep, can be accomplishing the important task of assessing what has happened, and help the individual come to terms with loss.

Dreams are considered to be an important means of working through emotionally charged experiences (Tatelbaum, 1981), and can play an important role in resolving grief. It is thought that useful grief therapy can be accomplished during sleep even when unpleasant dreams or nightmares are experienced. Alternatively, bereaved people may experience pleasant dreams of past times, which fulfil their desire for reunion, but result in bitter upset and disappointment on waking.

Talking about the significance and impact of troubled thoughts and dreams is important. This does not necessarily require detailed knowledge of the significance and interpretation of dreams; discussing them, and listening to how the individual feels about them, can be helpful in calming a restless mind.

Discussing troubled sleep patterns and dreams is important in reconciling the joint need for rest and recollection. Instead of troubled ideas and thoughts dominating the mind, preventing rest, talking can encourage the open expression of worries and fears, helping people place their thoughts and fears into perspective, and eventually come to terms with them.

Some older people, often with considerable encouragement, want to take sleeping drugs to encourage sleep. The role of antidepressant and sedative drugs should be limited; they should perhaps be used as a short-term expedient to obtain sleep after long periods of sleeplessness, but not as an alternative to individuals being allowed to 'feel' their pain. An over-reliance upon drugs can prevent this, delaying the process of recovery.

The maintenance of health

Human health is subject to a complicated variety of factors. Although bereavement is not an illness, and should not be considered as such, research is now confirming what general observation has long made us aware of:

that grief following significant loss frequently precedes the onset of illness, disease, and can lead to death.

Traumatic 'life events', particularly those which involve loss, have been found to be significant antecedents for a wide range of physical and mental illness. This controversial proposal made by Brown and Harris (1978) has been supported by subsequent research, indicating that bereavement is an important factor in the development of both physical and mental illness, often through its impact on the body's immune system.

The emotional turmoil surrounding grief has been found to produce a variety of physical symptoms; sometimes these may be identified with the final illness of the deceased. They include many general, nonspecific symptoms including:

- heart palpitations

- loss of appetite
- ringing in the ears
- digestive problems
- nausea
- dizziness
- nightmares
- constriction in the throat
- muscular pain
- impeded concentration
- poor memory
- insomnia.

Grief can provoke more serious physical or mental illness, particularly emotionally-based problems such as asthma, migraine, colitis, and arthritis, and many psychosomatic disorders. Such illness often complicates existing conditions or weaknesses rather than causing new health problems. Simonton *et al.* (1986) noted that stress increases susceptibility to illness by lowering resistance to infection through weakening the body's immune defence. They linked emotional factors, such as grief, with the onset of cancer, finding that prior to contracting the disease patients often recalled feeling hopeless, wishing for death, or seeing death as the only solution to their despair.

The problem of health is often exacerbated by self-neglect. Many grieving people believe that self-neglect is an essential part of manifesting grief. Such behaviour can also represent the search for sympathy and care, where social functioning deteriorates, and the individual seems less able to cope without considerable support.

Such an attitude needs to be countered; healthy grieving is founded upon self-care and self-worth.

There are also links between bereavement and mental health, first mooted by psychoanalysts in the late 19th century. It is important that the emotional distress caused by loss is not categorised as psychiatric illness. Yet the traumas of bereavement are difficult to manage, particularly for people who have previously been vulnerable to emotional ill-health. The inner conflict generated by significant loss can lead to changed, even anti-social, behaviour, dependency on alcohol or drugs, eating disorders, thoughts of suicide, anxiety states, phobias, behaviour disorders, or depressive illness, and this is particularly common when there is excessive guilt and self-reproach.

Significant loss also increases the risk of death. Modern medicine does not recognise that death can be caused by grief, or 'a broken heart'. Earlier medical practitioners did, and perhaps they were wiser. There is considerable evidence that the death rate during the six months following bereavement is significantly increased:

many older people just give up and die.

Such deaths may not result directly from bereavement, but from increased vulnerability to pre-existing illness, such as coronary thrombosis and arteriosclerotic heart disease, conditions that can be exacerbated by the emotional stress of bereavement.

Bereavement is, of course, closely associated with depression, which in turn can lead to thoughts of suicide. There is a higher risk of suicide in old age, and recent bereavement increases the risk.

Bereaved people need to be aware of the health dangers arising from their troubled emotions. It is common for older people to resort to an excessive consumption of coffee, tea, and other stimulants during the grieving period. These do nothing to help the process of recovery, and immoderate consumption can lead to the development of health problems in its own right (Scrutton, 1992).

There are simpler, more effective solutions. The importance of rest and sleep, healthy exercise, and good nutrition are all important, and carers should encourage these whenever possible.

Hope: the healing process

Older bereaved people have to deal with many difficulties before they are able to recover from loss and continue their lives.

Neither bereavement nor old age are considered times of optimism and hope. In combination they can prove to be devastatingly depressing.

Reduced self-esteem is characteristic of the mourning process. Significant loss can destroy self-confidence, and grief can deplete personal energy. This ensures that for many older people, bereavement can seem to be an entirely negative, hopeless, miserable experience. And this has to be added to ageist perceptions associated with their advancing years.

The result is that many bereaved older people believe that recovery from grief is impossible. If this feeling is not to become self-fulfilling it is vital that they are encouraged to feel more positively about the future.

Personal expectations, a willingness to recover, and the hope and expectation that recovery is possible, are essential ingredients to the process of recovery.

Older people need to work through their grief in order to overcome the combination of old age and significant loss, and to look positively towards the future. Grief will remain a negative, hopeless experience unless the individual, regardless of age, learns to use it positively. To achieve this, bereaved people need to be able to find meaning in their loss so that they can eventually transform their grief into something which supports future life.

Death is a natural life event. It is possible, and indeed vital, for older people to view personal death, and the death of loved ones, as an opportunity to develop emotionally. Such a process of growth involves:

- working towards a dignified death
- preparing for life without an important partner.

Both tasks are momentous, involving considerable pain and major life adjustment, but it is possible for older people to achieve both, and important that other people are prepared to assist them in the transition.

The willingness to permit grief to end is an important prerequisite to recovery. There is a powerful idea that the pain of loss is, or should be, never-ending, that sorrow is endless, that grieving is a sign of love for the deceased, and that it would dishonour the memory of the dead to return to a happy, fulfilling life.

Sometimes grieving people can become fully immersed in their grief, and it becomes necessary to examine the reason for their resistance to recovery. When faced with such intractable feelings, even a caring, supportive presence is insufficient, and carers can begin to feel inadequate. Then, the help offered to bereaved people needs to be more than a simple, caring presence, offering kindness and practical support. Carers will require more information on how to respond, and develop some skills with which to approach the problem.

Counselling skills can provide older bereaved people with the support and encouragement they need to use the bereavement experience as a stepping stone to personal growth, and a future which envisages satisfaction, achievement and growth.

4 A counselling approach to bereavement

Give Sorrow words; the grief that does not speak
knits up the o'erwrought heart and bids it break.
Shakespeare (Macbeth)

Counselling developed from the belief that the best way of healing the emotional distress people suffer is found within each individual (Carl Rogers, 1984). Each person has inner strengths and resources that can be utilised in self-healing, and recovery arises most effectively by helping people use their own unique abilities and experiences to this purpose.

Counselling skills are ideally suited to the problems of grief. This brief description of the role and principles of counselling examines how the techniques can be used at each stage of the mourning process.

Counselling techniques are not difficult to master, and those who wish to read more about the skills and techniques of counselling should refer to more detailed descriptions of bereavement counselling (notably, Worden, 1982; Raphael, 1984; Parkes, 1981b), and to texts dealing with counselling older people (Scrutton, 1989).

However, counselling older people through grief does depend crucially upon a capacity to see, embrace and transmit the importance of giving help to people regardless of their age, and regardless of their potential lifespan. Indeed when caring for the terminally ill, it depends on providing care right up to the point of death. To do this involves distinguishing between the quality, as opposed to the quantity of life available to an individual.

When working with older people, there is no need to deny the shortness of time that might be available to them; most older people have come to terms with this. What is more important is discovering how the time available can most profitably, and most enjoyably be spent by the individual.

The links between counselling and bereavement

The needs of bereaved people, and the purposes of counselling techniques are ideally matched, as the following table, which compares both, indicates.

Needs of the bereaved

- To be helped to understand, and come to terms with loss.

- To be helped to identify and express their personal feelings regarding loss.

- For an individual's sense of loss, to be understood and for an understanding to be reached of how this is likely to affect them, allowing for differences in personal needs and responses.

- To be offered support, and reassurance of their sanity, and help in interpreting 'normal' behaviour. People who may feel that they are 'going crazy', need reassurance that they will recover in time.

- To be given sufficient time and space for grief, and ultimately to reassess and redirect their future lives without the deceased.

Principles of counselling

- The primary purpose of counselling is to encourage self-expression; the counselling task is to encourage people to speak about their loss.

- Counselling focuses on feelings, and is specifically targeted at people who find it difficult, for whatever reason, to identify and express their feelings; this is particularly important when feelings affect their ability to live their lives.

- The object of counselling is to be person-centred, to focus exclusively on the problems as seen by the counsellee. Counselling techniques can therefore ensure that individual differences are accepted.

- The objective of counselling is to be *non-judgemental* towards the counsellee, and to offer them *unconditional positive regard*; this allows the counsellor to reassure bereaved people that their feelings and behaviour are 'normal' given the disruption in their lives.

- Counselling seeks to make people aware that there is someone prepared take the time, and a personal interest in how they feel, ensuring that all the worries, concerns, problems, and difficulties about the future are adequately discussed.

(Needs of the bereaved)

- To be given the opportunity, and the responsibility for making their own decisions about the future.

(Principles of counselling)

- Counselling is a 'non-directive' technique, which allows counsellees to reflect on their situation, to consider their options, and, in their own time, to make decisions about what they wish to do. Counselling is a 'problem solving' approach which seeks to identify the problems that loss has created, and then help people arrive at their own decisions and solutions to those problems.

- For emotional withdrawal from the deceased person to be facilitated.

- Counselling can encourage people to examine why they feel unable to redirect their energy away from the deceased, and help them to look at moving on towards investing in new situations and relationships.

- To be helped to examine how they are coping with their feelings. Those who are either refusing, or feel unable to redirect their lives successfully need to be challenged.

- Counselling seeks to understand how people try to minimise their pain, including the personal defence they construct to deny their feelings. Whilst understanding the reasons for this, it can challenge people who appear to be failing to cope, or who are resorting to denial, such as social withdrawal, drinking, or drugs.

Evaluation of bereavement counselling has indicated that it can reduce the damaging effects of bereavement, especially for those people deemed to be more at risk of poor outcome, where support is available soon after bereavement (Parkes and Weiss, 1983; Parkes, 1981a). It is therefore worth examining counselling techniques in more detail, in order to ascertain how they can be used in relation to older bereaved people.

The value of self-expression

The expression of grief seems to facilitate recovery from bereavement. The ability to share feelings with another person, to grieve together, and eventually to review and mourn the lost relationship are important to ensure that grief is neither avoided or repressed. Since Lindemann's classical paper (1944), poor recovery has been closely associated with the inhibition of grief, and it is increasingly recognised that successful recovery is difficult unless bereaved people can fully express their grief. Failure to do so can lead to higher mortality rates, and a greater incidence of mental instability.

Grief counselling seeks to ensure that bereaved people face their feelings openly and honestly, can tolerate the pain that this produces, and counselling also seeks to offer support for as long as it takes to recover. It is difficult to pass through bereavement without emotional distress; to deny, hide, or dull this pain in any way can result in its prolongation. It is important that bereaved people understand that it is acceptable to:

feel exactly what they feel

and to

express what they wish to express.

Personal grief should be experienced fully as this is what permits the individual to come to terms with loss, and eventually, to recover from it.

The process of experiencing emotional pain has within it the power to heal.

Yet openness is often difficult to achieve. There is fear of the intense emotions, especially the anger and acute distress which often accompany grief. Older people may have particular problems:

- some will have grown up within a social setting which frowned upon the open expression of grief, and which encouraged denial; they may be reluctant to grieve openly, and thereby prevented from moving towards recovery
- increased isolation, ill-health and financial problems may mean that some older people have less social support available to them for expressing their feelings
- and in older age there may be several, cumulative losses occurring over a relatively short time, reducing their social network, and making it more difficult to share their feelings with others.

To grieve fully demands enormous courage, particularly in a society that values emotional restraint, and where bereaved people risk disapproval for openly expressing their grief. In offering support it is important that feelings should not be avoided, and that pain is shared. In large measure, the skill of dealing with bereavement in its early stages is to help the individual understand that their emotional pain is real, and that it is acceptable to express it.

However painful the grieving process is, the cost of unexpressed, inhibited grief is known to be more serious. Some methods people use to avoid their feelings are:

- prolonged apathy
- a lack of desire for continued life
- withdrawal from active social involvement
- compulsive behaviour, overwork, over-busy-ness
- excessive drink or alcoholism
- reliance on prescribed medication
- constant illness and chronic physical symptoms
- a preoccupation with personal death, or suicide.

The initial counselling task should be to create a setting in which personal grief can be expressed, and within which the sorrow and hurt can be shared. Such a setting requires that the bereaved person:

- feels secure
- can express anger
- or just sit in silence.
- has permission to cry
- can reminisce

The expression of emotion within a counselling relationship should be neither encouraged nor discouraged. What is required is a natural rather than a forced expression of feeling, arising from open and honest discussion, and undertaken at the pace of the bereaved person.

The role of the counsellor is to help people acknowledge, and ultimately to come to terms with loss; it recognises the importance of feelings, and is specifically devised to enable self-expression; it seeks to identify real feelings, and to ensure that they are openly expressed.

Self-expression is important to both to men and women, but cultural role expectations can make it more difficult for men to discuss their feelings. Men tend not to have the same level or quality of peer support as women. Male friendship is often less aware of the value of intimate discussion at a 'feeling' level. Men are more practical, more task oriented; women tend more readily to form relationships based on emotional exchange and self-expression, and their bonds are generally stronger.

However, a word of caution is required. Whilst self-expression is a necessary prerequisite for recovery, it is not, on its own, sufficient.

It would be dangerous for counsellors to assume that if they have been successful in encouraging self-expression, and have perhaps induced tears, that the task of recovery is over (Parkes and Weiss, 1983). The counselling process has to move on from the expression of grief towards recovery, and the re-establishment of a new life.

Listening

Listening is the essence of counselling. The ability to listen precisely to what people say, and as important, to sense the feelings that lie beyond the words, are both vital to a full understanding of the individual.

Listening is particularly important in the early stages of mourning. Communication with bereaved people need not involve much talking by the counsellor, as this can sometimes inhibit self-expression:

- it is what the individual wants to say that is important
- for the counsellor, it is understanding what is being said that is important.

What remains unsaid can also be instructive, particularly as people in grief often find it difficult to express their feelings verbally. It is important to observe non-verbal messages, body language, and other indications of distress, pain, fear, and anger.

It is also important to recognise that when an individual finds verbal expression difficult it might be possible, and often more productive, to encourage them to write, draw or indeed to use any other 'artistic' means of expression. This does not necessarily have to involve skilful artistic expression; it is sufficient that the individual is encouraged to use the best, most comfortable medium to express feelings and thoughts accurately.

Staudacher (1988) indicates that writing can take many forms, depending upon the skills and interests of the individual:

- a farewell poem to a loved one
- an epitaph
- a description of deceased
- a life-story
- an expression of how important the deceased has been.

For many people with the skill to do so, drawing, painting and sculpture can express feelings more succinctly, and more accurately than any number of words.

A person-centred approach

Bereavement is a time when the needs and feelings of the individual are paramount. Counselling is a 'person-centred' approach, embodying the principles of:

beginning where the client is

and

moving at the client's pace.

Such an approach demands considerable patience, often when the counsellor can feel helpless and inadequate in the presence of painful grief.
Other agendas, notably the personal or professional needs of others
(including the counsellor) should be of secondary importance. Thus:

- the tendency to give advice or to reassure
- the desire to move bereaved people onward more quickly towards an
  acceptance of loss
- any impatience over the counsellee's apparent inability to progress
  towards recovery

should all be firmly restricted by the counsellor.

There is also a tendency to reassure when reassurance is not effective
or realistic. It is unhelpful to say:

'you will soon feel better' or 'things won't seem so bad in a few weeks'.

Life is as bad as it can be to the individual, and any attempt to avoid this
serves to minimise the significance of loss, and increase their sense of
isolation. To be person-centred requires that the counsellor seeks to
enable individuals to feel their pain and sorrow, and to understand and
accept feelings as they are.

A person-centred approach is beneficial in demonstrating that the
counsellor has their interests and feelings at the forefront of his/her
concern. This can be a considerable consolation, a form of reassurance
which does not rely upon, and is far more important than, giving them
meaningless, often self-defeating expressions of sympathy and understanding.

Of course, even for a 'person-centred' approach to be effective there
has to be a degree of acceptance by the bereaved person of the help being
offered. However well-intentioned, skilful, or compassionate the
approach taken, bereaved people may fail to benefit from the support
offered. Counselling cannot be forced upon an individual, and if the
wishes of the individual are to be paramount, such feelings have to be
considered.

A non-directive approach

The early stages of bereavement

Counsellors should not enter into a counselling relationship with the
intention of directing bereaved people to alter their attitudes, to change
their behaviour, or to control their emotions. Whilst this may be the
ultimate outcome of counselling, and might be in the best interests of the
counsellee, such movement should emanate from the individual.

It is not the task of the counsellor to advise, or tell people how they
should grieve, or to impose a timetable for their recovery.

This remains so even when the grieving individual wishes to be told what to do, when advice is actively sought, or when they ask for specific answers to their worries and concerns.

Many people will seek this type of directive support, but within a counselling approach it is important to ensure that decisions are taken by the individual. Such requests or questions are better answered indirectly through replies which seek to:

- draw from the counsellee their thoughts, feelings, and personal wishes
- outline and examine the range of options available to the individual
- support the individual in making a personal decision or choice from those options.

Question	Possible answer
• 'What should I do?'	• 'What do you feel you can do; or want to do?'
• 'What would you do in my position?'	• 'That is difficult because I do not know how you feel. Let's consider the choices you have.'
• 'Will I ever feel better?'	• 'Do you want to feel better? What can you do to feel better?'
• 'Do you think he/she would have wanted me to do this?'	• 'What do you believe she/he would have wanted you to do?'

The later stages of bereavement

Once the counselling relationship is firmly established, and the grieving process has moved on from the initial shock and pain, the emphasis of counselling can gradually move from its non-directive basis towards a more pro-active encouragement to move on. The counsellor can initiate discussion about what they need to do to assist recovery, to raise self-esteem, and move towards social reintegration.

The counsellor can assist the decision-making by establishing the tasks and objectives that are required in order to begin the process of making new life-choices, and re-establishing former life-patterns:

- 'Let us look at the areas in which you need to make decisions.'
- 'Let us look at the options that you have within each of these areas.'

In the early stages of grief, emotional attachment to the counsellor need not be discouraged as this can eventually provide the necessary security an individual requires for moving towards recovery. In the later stages, however, if the individual is clearly not emerging successfully from grief, or where the process towards recovery has become stuck, the counsellor has to consider the possibility that:

- an unhealthy or dependent relationship might be forming that is being inappropriately used by the bereaved person
- the counselling relationship is serving as a prop rather than as a means of personal recovery
- counselling support is being used to sustain the individual's desire to cling to the past, to retain their grief, and to withdraw from social life rather than to move towards social reintegration.

Where there is only limited movement towards recovery the counselling approach may need to be less non-directive, aiming instead at fostering and rewarding the development of self-help. Some movement towards personal autonomy can become a precondition for continued counselling support, with further support being offered on the understanding that it will be reduced or withdrawn when it is no longer needed (because recovery has happened), or if the person remains unwilling to move towards recovery.

Clearly, these judgements are complicated, and it is for these reasons that counsellors need to have personal support to help make them, or indeed, whether faced with such a situation they feel able to cope with the situation unaided. This will be considered in more detail in Chapter 6.

A non-judgemental attitude

The primary objective of the counsellor is to uncover feelings and attitudes. It is not to make judgements, or to form opinions about them. Emotions are what an individual feels, and at times of emotional distress the attitudes and behaviour which arise are often difficult to control, modify or change.

We all have opinions about how people should and should not respond to loss, opinions which arise from cultural understandings. The assumption that the coping process passes through distinct stages leads to people evaluating or 'judging' those who do not 'conform' to them appropriately. There are two main assumptions:

- that people should pass through a period of intense distress; failure to do so is thought to indicate a lack of sensitivity of feeling
- that people should recover after a relatively brief period of time, and return to normal levels of functioning as soon as possible.

We should seek to avoid such assumptions. The ability to be non-judgemental in the face of grief is important, particularly when the individual feels bitter and angry, or when they harbour levels of guilt and remorse which appear irrational. Faced with such reactions, the counsellor should remain as 'person-centred', 'value-free', and 'non-directive' as possible.

Judgements concerning the correctness, the rationality, the good sense of such matters, or any disapproval or condemnation of them, are neither helpful to the individual, nor the counselling relationship. Personal value judgements cannot change how another person feels: but they can create barriers which damage relationships, and prevent further constructive support arising from them.

Yet in the later stages of grief, it is not always possible, or helpful to be entirely non-judgemental:

- the counsellor may occasionally want to express personal reactions, something that is important within any genuine relationship (see the section on genuineness below)
- it may be necessary for the counsellor to suggest to bereaved people that their objective should be recovery, and a return to a satisfactory level of social reintegration
- bereaved people will often require someone who will not only provide approval, but praise for any progress made towards recovery.

Counsellors can help identify actions that are likely to be helpful, and others that might be damaging to recovery. Yet even here, the counsellor does not have to either agree or disagree, approve or disapprove, but assist in clarifying what they wish to do, and to discuss the advantages and disadvantages of taking any particular course of action.

Unconditional positive regard

The counsellor should seek to develop a positive, accepting attitude towards the bereaved individual, ensuring that the counselling relationship is based on mutual respect. We have seen how both old age and bereavement can undermine self-respect and confidence, and it is important for people to feel that they have our respect, as well as our unqualified attention.

Unconditional positive regard can indicate to people that they are worthy of such attention, that they are not regarded as inferior, foolish, or irrational because of the way they feel, or the way they are responding. In return, the counsellor can earn their respect and confidence, enhancing the effectiveness of the counselling relationship.

Unconditional positive regard also recognises that bereaved people, regardless of age, and however severe the loss suffered, have within themselves the inner resources for overcoming their problems and redirecting their lives. This has many implications for counsellors:

- they should believe that ageing bereaved people have an inherent dignity and worth, with a right to self-determination

- they have to rely upon the inherent capacity of the counsellee to choose their own values, attitudes and approach in the process of redirecting their lives
- that older bereaved people are able to achieve the necessary changes in their own self-interest.

Unconditional positive regard should apply in the most difficult situations, even when an individual has perhaps decided that life is no longer worthwhile, or where suicide or euthanasia are being actively considered.

Empathetic understanding

We cannot know for certain what is going on within the mind of another person. Nor can the counsellor assume that a particular insight is necessarily correct, or correct for any length of time. Despite this, it is important that the counsellor attempts to view the world

exactly as the bereaved person currently sees it

no matter how illogical, or irrational this impression may seem amidst grief-induced depression, anger and guilt.

An important part of listening is being able to sense what is being felt – empathy. Empathy is the capacity to 'feel' with another person, an attempt to enter their world of feeling as if it were our own, and to do so without the distancing effects of either fear or pity.

Only through empathy can the counsellor hope to understand some of the apparently foolish or self-damaging aspects of the social behaviour often displayed by grieving people (Scrutton, 1989). Empathy enables the counsellor to form tentative explanations or interpretations of what is happening in the life of another person:

- what they are thinking
- why they are thinking in that way
- linking this understanding with current social performance.

Empathy is more than pity, or even sympathy. Pity can patronise, placing a barrier between people. Sympathy implies a degree of compassion and sensitivity towards another person's situation, but without trying to understand it more deeply. Empathy involves an attempt to understand another person entirely: to climb into his/her shoes, to be sensitive to the way that person feels, to gain an understanding of why s/he is thinking and behaving in a particular way.

Empathy is a defence against resorting to banal reassurance. The counsellor needs to understand that:

- everything is 'not alright'
- that even if the pain will subside, current reality is painful.

Empathy requires that we explore and test the pain of grief:

- 'Tell me how it feels.'
- 'Tell me how you might deal with your pain.'

This may be a painful process for both parties, but it will not increase the suffering as is sometimes suggested. The pain already exists. The counsellor is merely asking for fuller understanding and clarification of the pain in order to offer support.

For the counsellor, the journey into pain is a necessary part of developing empathy – to understand, to seek, to share the feelings of a bereaved person. There are several 'levels' at which empathy can be attained:

- where empathy is non-existent: demonstrated by dismissive or denying remarks which indicate not only that we are not aware of how the other person is feeling, but are making no attempt to do so:

  'It was meant to happen; there's no explaining it; you need to cheer up; it's no use being morose; you are lucky compared to some people; everyone else copes with this kind of thing.'

- empathy that indicates some realisation that an individual's emotions have been affected, but without any attempt to find out how, or to what extent:

  'You must feel sad; it must have been a shock; I am sorry; is there anything I can do to help?'

- empathy that indicates an awareness of the individual's emotional state, alongside some attempt to develop understanding and link to personal experience:

  'You must feel sad; I remember when I lost … I felt so alone; do you feel the same?'

- empathy that indicates insight and observation into the feelings of the individual:

  'You must feel sad; you are not usually like this; perhaps you feel that life is no longer important to you; you seem to be angry, do you feel frightened about being alone?'

Empathy may precede a willingness to discuss deeper feelings. Initially people cannot express their emotions, although they are intensely felt. When to begin discussing them itself requires empathy. There needs to be an underlying basis of trust, which can take some time to build, before some people are willing to express fully their despair and anger.

To maintain empathy there is a continual need to test and re-test the assumptions that have been made, checking and updating where the bereaved person is at any moment of time. The changing nature of grief, the ups and downs of emotional life, ensure that the counsellor is not part of a static situation, but one in a constant state of flux. This can be done by 'reflecting back', perhaps by restating their own words, or finding our own words to interpret how we believe they feel, giving them an opportunity to agree or disagree with what you have said.

Genuineness

Genuineness, also called congruence, occurs when we can be real, or genuine, and do not make ourselves out to be something other than we are. The individual is aware of their inner feelings, and can accept themselves as they are, conveying this sense of self-acceptance to other people. Genuineness enables a more trusting relationship to develop.

Counselling should be a two-way process. The counsellor seeks to persuade the individual to speak honestly about themselves, revealing his/her own feelings, so in return the individual should be able to relate honestly to the counsellee. Counsellors should be prepared to share parts of themselves, to talk openly and honestly about the feelings and experiences they have in common, or indeed to share the pain of facing their grief. It can be useful to share personal experiences of loss, or indeed, to admit that they have not experienced the same kind of loss before.

It is often helpful for bereaved people to hear about the experience of those who have previously suffered loss. Sharing personal feelings and experiences can often indicate that people are not alone in their feelings, and that despite their current pain, recovery is possible. It offers bereaved people renewed hope of personal survival.

Openness has other rewards. People are more likely to share with those who are prepared to discuss their own feelings and weaknesses. For counsellors in a professional capacity – social workers, medical staff, clerics and others – concepts of 'professional distance' are unhelpful, implying an assumed superiority that can positively damage the counselling relationship. They have to work even harder at creating a relationship which is 'genuine'. Friends and relatives have a positive advantage over professional counsellors in this respect.

Trust and confidentiality

Trust is essential in any relationship requiring openness and honesty, particularly when dealing with the intimate emotional issues surrounding grief. Discussing the intimate details of life, if subsequently shared with other people, can lead to embarrassment, guilt or anxiety.

No-one reveals their deeper feelings to people they do not trust; we all require reassurance that the people who offer help are trustworthy. If doubt exists, perhaps through a lack of sympathy, a suggestion of intolerance or disingenuousness, or a feeling that someone has an ulterior motive in offering help, people will hold back from full disclosure of feeling. This is particularly so when dealing with people who, both by virtue of their loss, their grief, and their older age, may feel that they are becoming increasingly worthless, that they are becoming more dependent upon the care of other people, and that their personal value is limited.

In order to establish a counselling relationship based on trust, all the previous factors in the counselling relationship are necessary. Trust is won by:

- demonstrating real concern
- listening attentively
- being accepting and non-judgemental
- being realistically positive
- providing hope for the future.

Bereaved people need to know that the counsellor genuinely wants to understand, and can be trusted to honour their confidences. Confidentiality is an essential basis for trust. There must be an assurance that information shared will remain strictly confidential, that nothing will be passed on to other people without their full knowledge and agreement.

Some counselling approaches

Having considered the main principles of counselling, and before moving on to apply these to particular aspects and stages of work with older bereaved people, some approaches, methods and techniques that can be applied to bereavement work can be considered.

Reminiscence

Bereavement is a bewildering time, when the mind is trying to make sense of the world, often working with great intensity and speed to re-explore the past. It is quite normal for older bereaved people to be concerned with the past. For many, the past is often easier to speak about than the pain and sorrow of the present reality. It can contain cherished memories which provide some temporary solace from a hurtful present, and an unknown, or uncertain future.

Indeed, reminiscing increases with age, and is common with the very old. It represents a life-review, going over, making sense, and giving meaning to the good and bad experiences of the past. Memories of former losses, and how they survived them, may be a helpful part of the process. The object of reminiscence work is to help people describe their lives before loss, and to begin to distinguish between the past and the new and different reality, placing lost relationships and experiences firmly in the past.

Unfortunately, the opportunity reminiscence provides is too often lost because reflection, or dwelling on the past, is seen as meaningless and unimportant. The incessant, repetitive nature of painful reminiscence may seem to imply that individual is focusing too much on the past, and refusing to come to terms with the present. Reminiscence can also be painful to friends and relatives who themselves may not wish to be reminded of times and events associated with their own grief:

- 'It is morbid to continue brooding over the past; you should not dwell on it so much.'
- 'You should be thinking and planning for the future now.'

Older people have important memories they wish to share, but many people feel that in doing so they are causing unnecessary pain for themselves. Even treasured memories may be followed by bitter frustration over what was lost, wasted, or what cannot now be achieved, or the absence of a major partner who is no longer available to share them.

Where loss involves an ambivalent or problematic relationship, the individual may feel angry about 'wasted' time, or they may blame themselves for real and imagined faults. Reminiscence often involves having to listen to negative thoughts, perhaps negative attitudes towards the deceased, or dwelling on 'upsetting' aspects of past.

In other cases, memories may be idealised, a tendency to dwell only what was good, perhaps because of fear of being disloyal, or alienating friends and relatives. This can inhibit the expression of anger or guilt.

Despite these objections, reminiscence and life review in old age are important. It is only when the process of the life-review becomes stuck, when people begin to repeat the same thoughts and memories, that the process may be seen to be problematic. Yet for many people, repetition arises when they feel that no-one is listening, or interested. Where response to reminiscence is positive, obsessive repetition will usually decline quickly as the individual will have reviewed important memories, and their loss will often no longer appear as a continuous, oppressive tragedy to be denied or avoided.

Reminiscence provides the counsellor with an early basis for conversation, and an important means of communication which can lead to useful outcomes. In the days following bereavement, individuals may be preoccupied with the details of their loss, and may want to recount:

- the final illness, or accident
- the funeral
- visits from family and friends
- the life of the deceased

- memories of their relationship together
- their last encounter
- any unfinished business between them.

People can gradually be encouraged to move from specific, recent memories, working backwards in time, gradually recalling memories and events, both happy and sorrowful, from earlier life (Collick, 1982). Reminiscence can be intense and vivid, and this may bring sadness, regret, anger, futility, guilt, relief, but if mourning is progressing, more of the real memories, both positive and negative, the good and bad, the happy and the sad, will be recalled, and any ambivalence gradually unravelled:

- **when it uncovers sorrow:** the process of talking and crying arises, a natural and important means of helping the individual come to terms with painful feelings
- **when it uncovers happiness:** those times of joy, triumph, and quiet contentment, can be treasured, and stored away.

In the early stages, sadness may predominate – sadness for what can no longer be, for former loves and pleasures, even for dissatisfactions, angers and frustrations that the bereaved can never experience again. Reminiscence can help people recall these past events and conflicts, review them, and help them come to terms with their past. Counsellors can use reminiscence as part of their task of helping them cope with their grief. It can:

- give loss a wider perspective, and help bereaved people come to terms with their present reality
- place the deceased in the past, separate from the present
- help survivors explore the meaning and importance of former relationships, and discover what remains in terms of memories and memorabilia
- help re-establish a realistic picture of the deceased person, neither idealizing or denigrating their memory
- place former relationships in their proper context, a mixture of sorrows and joys.

Reminiscence can help people to allow the deceased to depart from the present, satisfied instead with keeping them 'alive' in the past, and in their memory. This sense of continuity can assist bereaved people in coming to terms with loss. It can help develop new insight into lost relationships. It can confirm that the essential nature and meaning of the lost relationship remains unchanged, part of a past they will continue to possess, and part of a new identity they are beginning to form.

Reminiscence can be used to help people cope with the anniversaries and other occasions that occur after loss; the opportunity can be taken to talk about their last Christmas, or their last holiday together, or the manner in which they used to celebrate birthdays and other occasions.

Old photographs and family mementos can be found and discussed, bringing considerable comfort to bereaved people. Opportunities can be taken to ask about interesting pictures, ornaments, joint activities or hobbies, all of which will be connected with shared experiences. These can form the basis of albums, and perhaps the starting point for writing a life-history, in prose or poetry, which can focus on the deceased, or their relationship together.

Many older people continue to suffer pain many years after bereavement, often because their grief has been suppressed, and recovery delayed as a result. Often, the reason for this was that no one was prepared to listen to them recalling their memories – reminiscence does require an audience. For these people, stuck in the mourning process, unable to relinquish their grief, it is possible to begin reminiscence work long after bereavement, and so belatedly begin the process of recovery.

The 'empty chair'

The empty chair is often used in Gestalt therapy. It seeks to change the normal one-to-one counselling situation by introducing the deceased, who is imagined to be sitting in the 'empty chair', providing an opportunity for an 'imaginary' conversation together where the bereaved person can talk about their thoughts and feelings concerning the loss of their relationship.

It can be a powerful technique, and one that most people accept readily when it is introduced spontaneously in discussion, and the reason for doing so is explained. The opportunity can arise when a person regrets not having done or said something to the deceased:

- 'If only I had told him I loved him.'
- 'I wish I could tell her how much I relied upon her.'

The counsellor can then suggest that they should use their imagination to do just that, that they should imagine that the deceased is in front of them, and that they should say whatever they want to say. The 'chair' is not essential. Often, a similar situation can be created by suggesting that the individual close their eyes, and imagine they are talking to the deceased. All painful feelings and thoughts can then be expressed, with the counsellor assisting and encouraging the process.

The dialogue is conducted aloud as this is believed to promote honesty, and enables individuals to listen to their inner feelings. It can be undertaken alone, or with a friend. It is an exercise that people will have to want to do, and can be difficult for many. The process can be difficult even for willing participants. It can produce various bodily sensations, including tears, shaking, dizziness, feelings of excessive heat or cold, which indicate that the person is reacting to the emotional intensity of the situation.

To be prepared for the exercise, the room should be set up privately and comfortably; time should be taken to breathe deeply and relax; the individual should be encouraged to concentrate their thoughts and feelings on the person sitting in the chair, which may have a photograph placed on it to help focus the mind.

It is a useful technique for resolving unfinished business, often a special concern for the survivors of tragedies, or following sudden or unexpected deaths, which may leave many regrets for things not said, or not done with the deceased. Counselling can enable the survivor to conclude this unfinished business, and find some way towards closure.

Reality testing

Bereaved people often struggle with personal guilt, especially following a sudden and unexpected bereavement. Such feelings are frequently expressed through 'If only ...' statements:

- 'If only I had done this.'
- 'Perhaps things would have turned out differently if I had said this.'

One important method of dealing with an individual who insists on feeling personally responsible or guilty for what has happened is to test the reality of such feelings. The counsellor should spend time discussing the issues of personal responsibility, and ask questions about whether anyone could really have changed what happened.

'Let us imagine that you had done this, how would that have made matters different?'

The benefit of reality testing is that the counsellor is not telling the individual that he/she is wrong – the latter is a more typical response which can create an argument in which the individual is obliged to maintain their position. Instead, the approach seeks to help the individual recognise that the event could not be avoided, and that they may not be personally culpable. Reality testing can also be usefully employed when an individual blames another person, a scapegoat, for what has happened.

The 'I want' exercise

The depression and low self-image that can arise in the vicious combination of old age and bereavement often leaves the individual feeling unimportant, unworthy and inconsequential. The individual can stop believing in the present or future, denying themselves the luxury of 'wanting'. This lack of hope and expectation can lock the individual in the past, and in a constant state of grief.

Everyone functions within self-imposed limits; ageism and grief ensure that many people place severe restrictions upon themselves and their expectations. These limitations need to be challenged so that people can permit themselves to develop and grow.

To overcome depression and grief, the 'I want' exercise seeks to enable people to have expectations, to make demands again, to assist in revitalising their life by helping them find a new sense of purpose and direction. It can help people review the possibilities that life can offer, and in doing so, help the individual reach out, expand and grow. Tatelbaum (1981) outlines several approaches to people commencing the exercise:

- to picture themselves as having the qualities they would need to enable them to do what they wanted
- to consider what they would be like, or what they would be doing, if they had the determination or courage (or some other quality) that was necessary
- to ask what a courageous (or strong) person would do to cope with their situation, perhaps someone they know, or might want to emulate.

Encouraging people to imagine themselves coping differently can help optimism and initiate change. It encourages people to move away from depressed modes of thought; it consider other ways of functioning; it enables the counsellor to ask whether they have the necessary qualities or characteristics to continue living; it can offer an individual a different scenario for future life, in which they might be able to play an active, helpful and fulfilling role.

Visualisation

Visualisation techniques encourage people to move way from grief and a restricted view of future life, and towards a broadened sense of self. Visualisations are pictures created in the imagination to help people change, or move away from a painful and difficult situation. The counsellor encourages the individual to picture, or visualise themselves:

- as they would want to be
- as if they had already undergone a process of change with all their wishes fulfilled.

Visualisation can function alongside techniques of meditation and relaxation, helping to establish a positive frame of mind from which to build imaginary, but desired pictures of the future. The aim is to motivate people to consider a more positive outlook, and through the imagination, to encourage self-motivation and the establishment of a new reality.

Changed perceptions can lead to changed perspectives about future life, encouraging the individual to take action to bring about what is desired, but which may appear distant. In this way, the individual can begin to see hope, and act on the basis that change is possible.

Group and family approaches

Although bereavement has been considered mainly in individual terms, it usually occurs within the context of family life. The family is a social system, distinguished by its wholeness, by the inter-relationship of its each members, and its relationship with the wider community.

There are various approaches to family work, all emphasising the importance of shared communication and feelings, of open discussion about the impact of loss, and recognising that people grieve, and adjust to loss, at different rates. Those who wish to discover more should consult the literature (for example, Whitaker, 1987; Masson, 1984; Treacher, 1984; Barker, 1992; Bowen, 1978; Lieberman, 1979).

A family focus has two main benefits. First, concentrating on an individual can impede or restrain the therapeutic value of family support in times of crisis. Second, an individual focus can imply that there is, or might be, a personal failure to cope with loss, and that grief demonstrates some form of weakness. Work with families should enable the expression of feelings, encouraging family members to respond to those who are in danger of becoming isolated, distressed or depressed. During mourning, it is important that the family is encouraged to share grief openly and honestly, and empathise with the pain each person is experiencing.

When people find it difficult to share their feelings and concerns, they may require the supportive presence of others; and such reserve is often best overcome within the family group. Some people may fear that their grief may upset others, or that expressing their pain may lead to the whole family system disintegrating in tears and distress.

The sharing of feelings and pain may involve many different experiences in the weeks and months following loss. A positive, supportive response can be a powerful confirmation of ongoing family affection and support. It can help overcome denial, facilitate an open review of the lost relationship, and encourage the process of recovery. When family members are able to communicate, to share information and decision making, there is an enhanced chance of good recovery following loss.

Family-based work following bereavement therefore provides an opportunity to construct wider networks of support for older people which should not be missed.

Yet difficulties may arise. Family work is based on the premise that it is a social unit in which all members interact and influence each other in ways which are broadly supportive. The well-integrated family can have a positive impact through its close, affectionate bonds which, in time of distress, can provide mutual and effective support within its ranks.

However, significant bereavement within a family can sometimes lead to the unit being unable to cope, incapable of offering support, or even becoming destructive. Indeed, the same family characteristics which enable the family to provide support in time of bereavement, not least its closeness, the sharing of resources, and the intimate knowledge of each other, can be the factors which, when negatively directed, can become injurious and disruptive. There are situations, particularly when supporting older people, where it will be difficult to work with the wider family, or where the family may hinder the grieving process:

- The family network may lose contact, live distantly, or become widely dispersed; the importance of family ties may have diminished by the demands of our modern, mobile society; many older people may feel emotionally separated from their family, with no role to play within it.
- A poorly integrated family may not be mutually supportive; for example, some dysfunctional families may need to have a scapegoat, someone who becomes the target for blame and anger following loss, often a weaker, more vulnerable member – sometimes an older person.
- The emotional trauma of loss may generate, or exacerbate divisions within the family, reducing its potential for support; the changes that loss brings can make the family unit dysfunctional, perhaps because the deceased played a key family role, or tensions arise when several family members feel that their loss is greatest, their pain worst, and their need for support and comfort pre-eminent.
- Family members may manifest grief differently, or at different times, thereby creating barriers; some may be unable to face the reality of loss, whilst others may have moved on to recovery.
- Families can vary widely in their ability to express and tolerate feelings; some may find it difficult to share their feelings and concerns; others may hide their grief in fear that it may cause further distress.
- The family may discount the significance of the loss, or act as if it has not happened – perhaps because the deceased was elderly.

So it is important to ascertain how the family might support or hinder emotional self-expression, so important to the recovery process. Do those most affected by the bereavement have the family's permission to express their feelings, fully and openly? Families which restrict emotional expression may prevent the resolution of grief, consequently making family-based work more difficult, although probably more necessary too.

For these reasons, bringing the family together to share in the grieving process may be daunting. However, whilst some families might be reluctant to enter formal meetings, informal settings, using times when the family usually meets together, can be used to encourage mutual support.

The social process of bereavement will often lead to changes in former roles, interactions, and communication patterns within the family. Each family contains within itself the various roles, pacts and alliances which determine the distribution of power, decision-making, mutual support, and the provision of self-esteem:

- the head of the family
- the sickly one
- the comedian
- the value setter
- the carer-nurturer
- the scapegoat.

Any loss within a family will affect the entire system. The death of one member can mean that former relationships, interactions, roles, communications, and needs can no longer be fulfilled in the same way. The death of a key family member can upset the family's equilibrium, creating the need to refill roles, make new alliances, and this can cause major tension and distress. Death is a crisis for family unit as well as for individuals.

The family's ability to reorganise role structures so that it continues to function can depend on the importance of the tasks previously fulfilled by the deceased. The reallocation of tasks requires flexibility, and those who seek to support the family have to understand such family dynamics in order to move it on so that it is capable of being supportive to its most bereaved members.

The lifeline

A major difficulty working with older bereaved people is the idea that they will not, and indeed cannot recover from their loss. Perhaps they feel too old, or too distressed to do so. The fact is, however, that the experience, strengths and skills that individuals possess are more important than age in the recovery process. One way of locating these personal qualities is 'the lifeline'. This exercise can be done on paper, along its length being drawn the person's lifeline:

Birth — 10 — 20 — 30 — 40 — 50 — 60 — 70 — 80

Above the line, significant losses and bereavements of the past can be listed – the loss of parents, other relatives, leaving home, marriage, retirement, and so on. Below the line, notes can be made about the significance of the event, whether happy or sad, how the individual felt about the event, responded to it, and eventually recovered from it.

Recognising how people recovered from previous loss will indicate how they may recover from current loss. Broadly, they will utilise the same personal characteristics:

- some will show resilience, others susceptibility to depression
- some will adapt, moving quickly on to develop a new life, others will become debilitated for some time.

Compared with this background life experience, we can assess more accurately how an individual is coping with the current situation. In doing so we can avoid the danger of making ageist assumptions about the chances of recovery, and how well or badly an individual is doing. Recovery is invariably more dependent on the coping abilities rather than the age of the individual, and this exercise can help make this point.

5 The recovery tasks

Bereavement may uncover many sensitive issues, the handling of which can require considerable skill. Research into bereavement has developed awareness of the stages through which grief can pass, its component parts, increasing our understanding of the process that bereaved people may have to pass on their way to recovery. Knowledge of these stages can be an important guide to what is happening in grief, and assist in deciding how best we can give support in any situation. An understanding of bereavement patterns should be used to enable carers to devise specific ways of responding to and supporting bereaved individuals.

Within each of the tasks outlined, the variety of emotional responses that may be faced will be considered, giving first an explanation of the specific emotion, followed by suggestions about how it can be managed, and the dangers of people becoming 'stuck', or 'blocked' at any point.

The bereavement tasks

Recovery from bereavement is a process which often starts from deepest despair, and moves on to the re-establishment of a new, reformed life pattern. This process involves change, much of it painful. No-one facing significant loss, least of all older people, can completely disregard their past and start life completely afresh. Recovery from bereavement involves recognizing that change has taken place, accepting the full implications of such change, re-examining former assumptions about the world and our role within it, all in order to continue living successfully.

This is a considerable journey. Worden (1982) outlines four tasks of mourning, which will be followed:

- to accept the reality of loss
- to experience the pain of grief
- to adjust to an environment without the deceased
- to withdraw emotional energy and reinvest in another relationship.

There is, however, an earlier task facing bereaved people which might be added: the task of 'preparing for bereavement'. This task is available to people who have time to anticipate and adjust to a potential or inevitable loss. It is not always available; but it is often available to older people, particularly older couples, and would be more so if the degree of social denial was widespread. Older people are closer to death than other generations, and could be given more encouragement to prepare for eventual loss.

Outlining the stages of bereavement assumes that people progress instinctively from one to another, and that if progress is disrupted in any way, supportive intervention aimed to work through the phases until recovery is complete, can help guide the individual towards more appropriate coping behaviour.

Yet in describing these stages, and what needs to be achieved in each, it is important to note that grief is not a stable, unchanging phenomenon, but a personal process within which there is continual change, development, and ultimately, personal growth. Each loss is unique, and each individual's response to loss is distinct.

Nor is there is a definitive schedule for recovery. The stages outlined serve as a useful guide, but a bad master; they should not be crudely superimposed upon individual experience of grief. There are inherent dangers in an inflexible understanding of the 'stages' of bereavement, when used to indicate that a valid, personal route is either inappropriate or wrong.

Nor should such categorisation presuppose that progress to recovery is uniform or straightforward, as each stage overlaps and blends together, with setbacks and regressions set against sudden advances.

Preparation for bereavement: secrecy or openness?

There is often a deep, impenetrable secrecy about the way that news of impending death is broken to both the dying, and their relatives and friends. Consequently, there is a continuing debate about the value of communicating openly about terminal illness.

Many professionals warn of the dangers of information, feeling that some people are not capable of accepting, or coming to terms with the prospect of death. They encourage families to withhold information on the basis that it might cause anxiety and needless emotional pain. Often such decisions are made on an assumption that the decision is concerned with the treatment of an individual's physical condition – however, they usually ignore the need to support the emotional needs of dying people, and the grief of close relatives and friends.

Many relatives and friends endorse the decision, often on no firmer basis than respect for professional opinion. Giving bad news is an experience that most people find difficult, perhaps not so much in the telling, but in coping with the reaction that might follow, and the emotional stress of witnessing the grief of bereaved people.

The benefits of preparing for bereavement

The idea that openness is valuable in dealing with inevitable, or actual loss is relatively new. The process started with Lindemann (1944) who concluded that bereaved people need to be encouraged to express rather than deny their feelings. More recent experience suggests that when anticipatory mourning is possible, with family and friends sharing their feelings with dying individuals, grief can be more bearable. There is now considerable evidence that pre-warning is not only tolerable, but ultimately beneficial to recovery. This is true in all kinds of loss:

● when people face a limb amputation
● when crippled patients refuse to accept a wheelchair
● when older people have to leave their homes
● when seriously ill patients refuse a life-saving operation.

In such situations, time is required before an individual is asked to make final decisions, and even they may require support to help express feelings.

Initially, bad news may create worry and anxiety; but this initial distress ultimately assists coming to terms with loss. Anticipating the limits and potential of life following loss, assisted by full, realistic information, eventually makes the period of mourning shorter and less severe, and the process of adjustment to the new reality easier to accept (Parkes, 1975).

An open approach, although initially difficult, has been found to offer comfort and peace to all concerned, and to play an important part in reducing the difficulties faced in the bereavement process. The hospice movement, which provides small hospitals for dying people, functions on the basis of openness and honesty about death, thereby enabling the family to prepare by:

● talking
● sharing feelings
● making arrangements
● saying final farewells.

The reverse is also true. Those who suffer sudden or unexpected loss have been found to have more difficulty coping than those who have been able to anticipate loss. Forewarning has several benefits which can help make significant loss an understandable, if undesired process:

● it can help people live with the prospect of loss, so that when it eventually occurs it is not unexpected

- it can help people make plans so that the task of living after loss is not felt to be a betrayal of the deceased.

For older people, anticipation is particularly important. They are often more aware of death so it is particularly foolish to shield them from bad news. It is important for us all to accept that human life is transient, that we need to prepare ourselves for loss, and to believe that there are ongoing sources of potential satisfaction and fulfilment available to us, even in old age.

Moreover, attempts to withhold information can lead to spiralling dishonesty, imposing intolerable burdens on many older people whose relationships may have endured for many years on the basis of honesty. Most older people will already understand the imminence of loss; and most people will prefer and appreciate being openly and honestly informed.

Yet whilst ageing makes open preparation especially apt, it also has inherent problems:

Will preparing older people for 'inevitable loss' make them too accepting, and become self-fulfilling?

There are, after all, times to resist and fight, as well as times to accept graciously what is inevitable. It is the difference between recognising:

- the unavoidable organic process of birth, renewal, decline and death

  and the medicalized concept of clinging on to life at all costs

- the ageist concept of the inevitability of pain, suffering and loss in old age

  and the insistence on maintaining optimism and normal functioning for as long as possible.

Will people prefer to postpone for as long as possible the pain of recognising, talking about, and planning for the significance of imminent loss?

It may seem natural for families to remain optimistic. Life is precious, even in face of painful terminal disease, and often both the dying and bereaved will hold strongly to hope and life whilst it remains. Yet this can make it difficult to acknowledge the imminence of loss. Even if the anticipation of loss is ultimately helpful, it is often difficult to persuade people to embark on the process prior to the event; to do so may appear to be disloyal to those still living, or to allow, even or 'invite' an event that we would rather not happen.

The truth should not normally be hidden. More energy should be utilised in finding sensitive ways of giving information, and subsequently supporting bereaved people than supporting an untruth. The task for those facing loss is to make as much use of the remaining time as possible: this cannot happen unless people are aware of what is likely to happen. Shielding people from the facts of life and death is not only unfair, it denies people the right to begin the grieving process, and encourages avoidance and denial.

Moreover, it is clear that counselling prior to an expected bereavement can be helpful to both individuals and families (Parkes and Weiss, 1983; Cameron and Parkes, 1983). When dying people and close friends have been able to accept death, sharing their deepest feelings, they are able to maximise the remaining time they have available, and together work through some of the problems that arise during the mourning period.

The ability to anticipate loss can reduce the shock and disable the impact of the event, assisting in recovery. Adequate preparation does not entirely prevent the trauma of loss; the painful process of grieving has to run its course; but anticipation can reduce feelings of bewilderment, improve the ability to grasp the event, and the acceptance of a world in which such capricious and gratuitous tragedies can occur.

Sharing information

Personal involvement is a key factor in the eventual acceptance of loss. If people have an opportunity to prepare themselves for loss then it should be encouraged. This means that realistic information, given as sensitively as possible, is required. It is then important to confirm that the information has been properly understood, and that support is offered to help them come to terms with impending loss.

This is not an easy task; feelings of fear and uncertainty about what to say at such times can sometimes ensure that communication can easily break down. Too often, insufficient emotional support is given to ensure that people are not overwhelmed by the news. Those who have to provide difficult information need to consider six factors:

1. Who should break the news? Should it be given directly to the person who will suffer the greatest loss? Or is there a relative or friend better placed to pass the information sensitively?
2. Information should be given through personal contact, and within a setting which is comfortable, private and safe.
3. It is wise to check what people already know, which is often more than is assumed. This can simplify the task, and allow more time for clarification and support.
4. The task takes time. People need to assimilate the news, react to it, and ask questions. Time needs to be taken to discover what has been understood, how it has been interpreted, and for clarification. Many mistakes can be made:

   - too little information can lead to misunderstanding
   - too much information can be confusing

- information given too soon may be incorrect
- late information may leave insufficient time.

5. The news should be given in simple, easily understood language which is specific, free from euphemism, and to the point. This avoids the possibility of misinterpretation. Bad news remains bad news however it is explained. There is no form of words which can reduce the pain; sensitivity is shown by our demeanour and attitude, not by stuttering, searching for the right word or phrase, embarrassment and beating around the bush.
6. The bearers of bad news have to be prepared to face the immediate emotional responses of the recipients, ranging from shock, denial, distress, anger, guilt, remorse and fear.

Anticipatory grief

Many deaths can be anticipated. With older people they can arise from a gradual decline in health and body function, or from disease and system failure. A period of anticipation can allow survivors to begin the task of mourning, and begin to experience the pain of loss. There has been much debate about whether people are able to grieve and come to terms with loss prior to the event. Gerber (1974) suggests that relatives of a dying patient may be able to use the terminal phase to plan for the time when they will be bereaved, that anticipation can be seen as a period of socialisation into the bereaved role.

Yet even though death may be anticipated, it will not prevent separation anxiety, or the resulting distress. Some deaths, even those considered to be 'timely', may remain 'unexpected' when they happen, and even anticipated death can produce severe grief. Indeed anticipation can intensify and prolong the separation process, and many problems may arise:

- the period of prolonged grieving can produce resentment, particularly when someone is dying of a slow, wasting illness – and harbouring such feelings can ultimately lead to guilt
- it can lead to survivors withdrawing from emotional involvement with the dying person too soon, again forming a later the basis for regret and guilt
- watching someone die can increase an awareness of personal mortality, and develop an anxiety about our own fate.

Dying people also experience anticipatory grief. Whilst survivors are losing one person, the dying individual is losing everyone. This can be an overwhelming experience which can take time to recognise and accept. Yet anticipation can enable sharing of the situation, giving comfort, support, companionship, and reassurance. It remains a difficult time, but

anticipation can intensify attachment, and encourage closeness and tenderness. There are many positive exercises that can help dying people
come to terms with personal death:

- discussing/writing their eulogy (how they would like to be
  remembered)
- discussing/writing their life-history
- discussing what they would wish to happen to those they leave
  behind.

Survivors also have an opportunity of preparing themselves for life
without the deceased. Anticipation may raise questions such as:

- 'What will I do?'
- 'Where will I live?'
- 'How will I manage?'

The time preceding loss can be used to rehearse such questions and can
be helpful in reducing the impact of subsequent grief, and to complete
unfinished business, whether financial, social or emotional, prior to
death. Key family members and friends can be encouraged to express
their feelings and thoughts; their appreciation and disappointments;
their hopes and fears; and many other matters that may usefully be
discussed before death.

When people are able to express regrets, make restitution for past acts
or omissions, and generally to conclude their relationship, it can help
avoid later anger, guilt or self-reproach, and survivors do not have to
grieve about what should have been done when they had the opportunity.

This is in marked contrast to people faced with sudden, unexpected
death, who often feel that they were denied time to say goodbye, to make
restitution for faults, to resolve quarrels, and to reconsider plans.

Using the time: commissions

Old age is never a time to put off until tomorrow things that can be done
today. The view that ageing people have 'time to kill' is ageist; and those
older people who live as if this is so have internalised dominant social
attitudes. The economic 'law of diminishing returns' informs us that the
rarer the commodity, the more valuable it becomes, and the more carefully it should be used.

As people grow older the more precious time becomes. This is particularly so for older people facing loss. Knowledge of imminent loss
intensifies rather than weakens the value of time, and the use to which it
should be put. When people are facing the end of a long relationship, it is
time to finalise many matters:

- to reminisce, to remind each other of shared experiences over the years
- to say 'thank you' for the things they have done together

- to apologise for the things that should have been done, but which remain undone or unfinished
- to say goodbye.

For the dying time can be used to discuss their fears, hopes and expectations; to discuss the hereafter; to discuss funeral arrangements, and any other matters of concern which helps them prepare for leaving the world.

For survivors time can be used to discuss the future, the decisions that have to be made, and the challenges and changes that will arise from bereavement.

Yet time can be used for more than this. It can be extremely helpful if dying people prior to death are able to discuss their hopes and expectations for those they leave behind. 'Deathbed commissions', made to close loving relatives, can have enormous force. They are made when dying people give 'permission' to survivors to act in certain ways after their death. Thoughtful, liberating commissions can make it clear that survivors should consider themselves free to re-establish their lives. This can create firm foundations for recovery from grief, recommencing life, and enable the individual to establish a new identity, entirely free from any feelings of guilt about disloyalty.

Alternatively, commissions can be binding, laying down expectations about the way survivors should conduct themselves in future. These can add considerably to the burden of bereavement.

Liberating commissions

- to unreservedly exonerate their partners from any blame for the death
- to thank the survivor for contributing to their happiness during their relationship
- to express the wish that survivors recommence their lives fully after death
- to give permission to form new relationships.

Binding commissions

- to express doubts or dissatisfaction about how death has happened
- to criticise the relationship, leaving doubts about the survivor's contributions
- to place restrictions on a survivor about what should and should not be done
- to show jealousy or express disapproval of a partner forming new relationships.

Commissions are not always expressed. Many expectations develop within relationships over time, even though they are implicit rather than explicit. Moreover, survivors can sometimes form unrealistic ideas, often based on ideas of fidelity, faithfulness, fealty and loyalty, about what their former partners would, and would not want them to do. Such expectations may or may not be accurate, but either way they can be powerful determinants of future behaviour, restraining freedom of action, restricting a survivor's ability to move through grief, and to re-establish a new identity. Checking on the accuracy and reasonableness of such implicit or explicit expectations through discussion can be important, particularly if it can be undertaken prior to bereavement.

Task 1: intellectual acceptance of bereavement

Loss, especially death, may be recognised but not accepted. The first task to be accomplished during the mourning period is to acknowledge and accept the new reality: that significant loss has occurred, and that important aspects of former life, have ended forever.

Many factors prevent people accepting the reality of loss. When someone dies, even if death was expected, it is difficult to accept that it has happened. Although death is a natural part of living, and everyone will die in time, we often view death as unimaginable, an outrage, an enemy to be defeated. Such denial is an intellectual deception; we all know that immortality is impossible, but we often live more in hope and expectation than in reality. This often gives rise to searching behaviour, to hallucinations, and to mis-identifying people with the deceased person.

This 'intellectual' denial of death is often assisted and sustained by the removal of death from public view; death is now confined to hospitals, nursing homes, mortuaries and funeral parlours, making the eventual reality of death more frightening than it needs to be.

The role of counselling in this initial task is to facilitate acceptance of what has occurred, to face reality:

- the individual is dead
- reunion is not possible.

It is not part of the counselling role to offer hope where none exists, to allow an individual to believe that what has happened has not taken place, that something which cannot be undone can be undone, or that the future can remain unchanged, unaltered.

In the early days of bereavement, the counsellor does not need to stress the point. The mechanism of shock, denial, and anger will prevent the full reality being too urgently enforced on the mind; any attempt to do so will be resisted, and can be counter-productive to the counselling relationship. Yet rather than connive with denial, the counsellor can gently respond to remarks which indicate disbelief by comments designed to reinforce the reality of what has happened.

Remark	Response
• 'I cannot believe that it has happened, I will wake up soon from this nightmare.'	• 'I can understand that it must be hard to take in what has happened at present.'

Later, responses can be firmer, indicating not only that the bereavement is a reality, but that it brings with it the need to change, and to rebuild a life which has been significantly changed.

- 'Yes, I can understand that it is difficult to come to terms with ... have you thought about what you feel you can do about it now?'

Encouraging the discussion of options and choices is an important method of moving conversation towards an acceptance of reality. It helps to move the individual from denial to practical considerations about future life, and enables the counsellor to assist bereaved people to look more optimistically at the future.

Shock and numbness

The period immediately following bereavement, particularly a sudden or unexpected death, is often one of great shock. Many bereaved people remember little of the days following significant loss, instead experiencing a feeling of numbness that can last for hours, days, and sometimes weeks.

Shock, and the numbness it creates, is a psychological defence mechanism which serves to block feelings and sensations that would otherwise be overwhelmingly painful, insulating the individual from the immediate intensity of pain and grief. People can appear to live in a state of unreality, only hazily aware of others around them. The same behaviour has been seen following major disasters – a lack of emotion, docility, unresponsiveness.

Numbness allows the mind to discount the full enormity and significance of loss, and the emotional crisis being faced. Afterwards, it is a time people often find hard to describe; it constitutes a kind of 'non-feeling', a sense of distance and isolation from events around them. It has been described as an unreal, dream-like state, during which the individual feels personally disengaged and isolated.

Sometimes, desensitisation can be so powerful that an individual cannot recall events, or their sequence. This can be particularly significant when working with older people, for it can, and often does lead to fears, even assumptions about possible senility. Provided that the grieving process is handled properly, this is not so; numbness is a normal response to loss and has no long-term effects on the mind.

If carers do not understand this mechanism, it can be perplexing. Bereaved people, who might be expected to be distraught, can sometimes appear superficially impassive and unruffled. Some people will make themselves busy with practical tasks, a way of avoiding the need to think about the significance of their loss. Others will become listless, lacking in energy. Their imperturbability might make it appear that they are coping with loss without emotion. Indeed, this is so. People in shock do not immediately recognise the full impact of what has happened, and therefore they are not yet grieving.

It is important to note that people differ in their initial reaction to loss. Stoical behaviour is, for some, a normal way of functioning – an attempt to reassure those around that they are coping with the impact of loss. For a short period, it can be accepted as such. Yet there are dangers when people do not move out of the initial 'shock' reaction to bereavement, and begin to feel pain.

With other people, the mind can alternate between being active and busy – and feeling entirely blank, unable to concentrate. Often, the individual will interact and respond to other people – whilst at other times feel unable to respond at all.

Some people will not experience shock or numbness, moving straight to the next, more painful stage of coming to terms with loss.

In the early post-bereavement period, carers need to accept shock and numbness, recognising it as a means of survival, a normal reaction to significant loss, temporarily rendering the individual incapable of dealing with people and decisions. It should not be rushed or hurried; even counselling cannot begin when people are in shock, and unable to discuss their feelings.

Any activities or decisions are often undertaken by carers during this time, providing them with purposeful activity for which they are often thankful. Indeed, carers may need to offer help pro-actively, as the state of numbness can prevent people asking for help.

The tranquillising effect of shock and numbness is temporary. Gradually, the mind is allowed to come to terms with what has happened. Soon the individual will re-emerge, experience pain, and begin to make demands on close friends and carers.

Distancing

Distancing is another defence mechanism evident during the early stages of grief. Again it is entirely compatible with eventual recovery. It is often achieved by bereaved people engrossing themselves in routine, monotonous activity, such as housework, which effectively redirects their attention away from loss, and the emotions which would otherwise result.

Distancing enables people to obtain relief from the intense pain produced by loss. They seek to detach themselves from what is happening, creating instead an illusion of a separate, insulated world within which they feel able to cope without going mad. Activity is used to fill the void left by loss, to stave off the yearning, sadness and pain which they would otherwise find too hard to bear.

It is difficult for carers to cope with. Distancing can create a sense of unreality, as people behave as though they are no longer involved in what is going on. They are difficult to communicate with, or to engage in any meaningful way. They require patient support and understanding, and it is important that they should be encouraged, although not forced, to emerge slowly from their self-imposed isolation.

Denial

'Mankind cannot bear too much reality.' TS Eliot

Denial is an advanced form of distancing, a refusal to accept loss, another psychological mechanism which enables people to refuse a too difficult reality. In this sense, it helps to protect the mind, a healthy way of blocking out painful thoughts and feelings, and keeping anxiety levels and stress to manageable limits. It is also a desperate means of self-defence, offering the individual a means of maintaining sanity. When faced with a sudden, massive loss, people can feel that the situation they face is so painful, unacceptable, and overwhelming that they cannot admit its reality. They will deny the chaos that has been introduced into their lives.

Denial is a normal response during the early stages of bereavement; the individual knows the reality, but has redirected attention away from their pain in order to gain temporary respite. This refusal to accept a new reality will eventually decline. People begin to experience the pain associated with loss, a fuller awareness of loss begins to emerge, although the mind may only gradually accept fully what has happened, and bear the resulting pain.

During the initial days of bereavement, the individual can cling to the belief that the loss has not occurred. With older bereaved people, denial can also be an attempt to avoid the painful recognition of personal mortality, and the approach of their own, ultimate loss.

Denial can provide temporary comfort, which may involve the individual searching for the deceased, sometimes sensing an invisible presence, whether this be a scent, a noise, a feeling or a touch. Denial can vary, but Dorpat (1973) has outlined three forms:

- denial of the facts of loss, ranging from slight distortion, to examples of full-blown delusion, for example, where a dead body has been kept un-notified in the house for weeks
- denial of the meaning of loss, in which people interpret loss as less significant than it is, perhaps by minimising the importance of the former relationship
- denying the irreversibility of the loss, refusing to believe that death has occurred, or believing that reunion is possible, perhaps through the medium of spiritualists.

It is important for counsellors to recognise that bereavement is a miserable experience, and that in the early days the emotional pain may seem unbearable to bereaved people. Yet it is also important to remember that all emotional pain is bearable, and ultimately self-limiting. The mind is initially 'closed down' through shock, whilst later experience of too much pain will cause anger, depression, or other forms of temporary self-protection. Bereaved people can be helped if they understand the process of recovery, and whilst this is not always immediately possible amidst current misery, it is the prospect of recovery that should always be kept in mind by the counsellor.

The counsellor should not collude with denial, and should try to keep the individual focused on loss. There are four lines of conversation that can help the individual talk about loss:

- 'Tell me a little about the death? What happened during that day?'
- 'Tell me about your relationship together? How did you meet?'
- 'Tell me about what has happened since the death? How have people been towards you?'
- 'Is this the worst loss you have suffered? Have you been through other times as bad as this? What did you do then?'

These topics can be introduced to gain an initial response, and to demonstrate that you are taking a personal interest, and are prepared to talk about matters, however difficult they might be.

Within a few weeks of bereavement, grief usually becomes less intense, and denial is no longer required. If it continues, however, it signifies that the individual is in danger of becoming 'stuck' in the grieving process. Persistent denial becomes a problem, signifying a frame of mind refusing to come to terms with the new reality, and is incompatible with recovery.

Continued denial neither prevents pain, nor assists recovery. Instead, other emotional reactions develop, such as anxiety and guilt, which indicate that the individual is grieving but refusing to accept loss. Action needs to be taken to get behind denial at this stage.

Every opportunity should be taken to focus grieving people on their loss, perhaps by talking about the deceased, using unreservedly words associated with death, to encourage viewing of the body, attending the funeral, or visiting the grave.

Searching

Another important early stage of the mourning process is the search for reunion. For many weeks people can continue to imagine the presence of the deceased:

- making meals and drinks
- searching faces in the street, and imagined sightings

- listening for sounds
- waiting for doors to open
- imagining noises associated with the deceased
- talking as if the deceased were still present
- calling out for the deceased person.

This searching behaviour can be very real for many people. For some, it can bring temporary comfort and peace; for others it can be deeply distressing. Yet regardless of the impact, searching is a normal reaction to losing something important, not only to death, but in other painful separations, and it can play a role in the early stages of bereavement.

Moreover, failure to find it makes us angry for being careless, for the inconvenience, or with other people for removing it. Parkes (1972) states:

'In social animals, from the earliest years, the principal behaviour pattern evoked by loss is searching.'

Lorenz (1963) described searching behaviour following the separation of a greylag goose from its mate, concluding that all the observable characteristics of the goose's behaviour were roughly identical with human grief:

'The first response to the disappearance of the partner consists in the anxious attempt to find him again. The goose moves about restlessly by day and night, flying great distances and visiting places where the partner might be found, uttering all the time the penetrating trisyllabic long-distance call …. The searching expeditions are extended farther and farther and quite often the searcher itself gets lost, or succumbs to an accident … .'

Anthropologists have studied the reaction to the loss of close relationships in different societies and cultures, discovering that searching behaviour is universal, often allied with the belief that in an afterlife there can be reunion.

Searching behaviour is thus both strange and understandable. When bereaved people search agitatedly for what they have lost, people often find it difficult to understand. The counselling task is to:

- offer reassurance that searching is normal
- confirm that the individual is not irrational, or unusual
- explain that searching is a phase which, in time, will pass.

Many older people feel quite unable to control their searching, or they feel frustrated when they fail to find what they know has gone. The problem of searching behaviour is clear; the dead are not available to find.

One danger is that older bereaved people will not discuss this behaviour. It can be worrying, leading to feelings of distress, foolishness, and bewilderment, particularly for older people who may fear losing control of their minds and the possibility of mental instability or dementia.

When the link between loss and searching is understood, older people are often relieved to know that their behaviour is normal. This alone may not end searching behaviour; but it can relieve the mental distress that can arise from it.

Many people faced with significant loss seek the assistance of spiritualists in their search, people who claim an ability to provide a 'medium' between the living and the dead. Whilst Spiritualism claims to help bereaved persons in their search for the dead, Parkes (1972) tested this and found that most people did not feel satisfied with the experience, with few continuing with regular attendance at spiritualist meetings.

Idealisation

Idealisation is a way of protecting ourselves from recognising difficulties that existed with a relationship. The tendency to idealise is strong, transforming the deceased person into someone more exceptional than in real life, disregarding factors that may once have exasperated and irritated. This focus on positive rather than realistic memories makes it possible to deny uncomfortable feelings of resentment, ambivalence, anger and guilt:

- to see perfection where in life there was imperfection
- to focus on good rather than bad characteristics
- to recall happy rather than unhappy times.

Those who had an ambivalent relationship with the deceased will often seek to idealise them after their death. This denies the real nature of the relationship, and such a reaction is often based on guilt. It is too late to apologise; there is no hope of restitution or forgiveness. Whilst the relationship continued, however painful, there was at least the prospect of reconciliation; now there is no chance to correct wrongs. Only guilt and unfinished business remain.

There is a tendency to feel that idealisation is at worst harmless, and at best a sign of constancy and faithfulness to the dead. It is, however, another form of grief avoidance, a form of denial which makes coping with loss harder, and recovery more difficult. If it persists, it indicates a reluctance to come to terms with death, a feature of unsuccessful grief.

Idealisation affects recovery from bereavement by establishing additional problems to readjustment:

- it makes the barrenness of the new reality worse than it is, or should be
- cherishing an illusion can prevent the formation of new relationships, either because they remain unwanted, or because of the difficulty other people have in measuring up to the idealised image.

Prolonged idealisation can happen when loss occurs to people who have difficulty in expressing their feelings. It can prevent moving on from grief. Yet if an individual has been capable of developing a 'special' relationship, they are capable of establishing another. Idealisation needs to be carefully challenged by the counsellor, perhaps by embarking on a 'reality testing' exercise:

- 'You seem to be indicating that he was a saint; almost super-human. It must have been difficult living with a saint! Did he have bad points?'
- 'Whenever I suggest that you may have angry/guilty feelings about her I notice that you do not want to consider them. Why do you think this is?'

Vilification

Vilification is the opposite of idealisation, and is also a protection against distressing grief. It seeks to deny the significance of the loss by undermining its importance. As with idealisation, the counsellor can 'reality test' in order to obtain a more accurate picture of the feelings of the bereaved individual:

- 'You seem to be seeing her as all bad. Perhaps you are unable to see her positive side because you are protecting yourself from accepting that you have lost something you valued and loved?'

Mummification

In relation to bereavement, the process of 'mummification' is connected with an unwillingness to move material possessions belonging to, or associated with the deceased. Instead, they are maintained in a `mummified' state, as if they are being kept for use when he/she is rediscovered. Many bereaved people wish to preserve their environment as it was when death occurred; Queen Victoria's reaction to the loss of Prince Albert can be cited as an example of this behaviour, part of the refusal to accept loss (Gorer, 1965).

Other bereaved people actually jettison clothes and other personal items that serve as an uncomfortable reminder of the deceased. This is the opposite of mummification, a reaction which seeks protection from pain by removing artifacts that would otherwise serve to remind them of their loss.

Both reactions indicate an inability to cope with loss by refusing to place former relationships into perspective, and in the past. A counselling approach should be neutral on both issues, neither encouraging or discouraging the removal or maintenance of belongings (although disposal of belongings is more irredeemable, and caution can be advised before 'final' decisions are taken).

The solution to mummification is to be found in helping the individual come to terms with loss; and this is not done in relation to either the disposal or retention of physical objects.

Conclusion

Intellectual acceptance can be considered to have taken place when three conditions are fulfilled:

- there is an absence of distortion, for example, where there is no expectation of return, or any continuing difficulty in believing the death has occurred, and no undue idealisation or denigration of the deceased
- the individual is able to remember and talk about their loss, although doing so may be uncomfortable and distressing
- where loss is integrated into their new reality, where the individual has accepted what has happened to them – although the pain remains.

Task two: emotional acceptance of bereavement

The second task of mourning begins when bereaved people start to experience the full impact of emotional distress that loss generates. The task is closely entwined with intellectual acceptance, but usually follows on from it. It is perhaps the most vital stage in the process of recovery from bereavement.

People can avoid emotional acceptance by cutting off their feelings, and denying their pain in all the ways that have been outlined. Such behaviour seeks to avoid having to think about personal pain, feeling it, and coming to terms with what has happened. The ability to express personal grief, rather than evading it, is an important element of recovery requiring that the bereaved person is able to spend time talking about their grief. To facilitate self-expression two requirements are necessary:

- suitable surroundings, quiet and free from activity, a setting where the grieving person feels safe, usually in the home of the bereaved individual
- the availability of caring people, willing to spend time listening to them, and to discuss their grief.

The feelings that need to be expressed will be considered later. Yet it is always easier to discuss practical issues, or to discuss emotional matters at an intellectual, rather than a 'feeling' level. This must be avoided. Counselling should be feeling-centred, responding to what people say by exploring further into the emotional content, and how the individual can cope with it.

Throughout the process, the counsellor needs to discuss emotional distress realistically, always acknowledging the significance of loss, but at the same time retaining a positive outlook on the longer-term situation, with a view to recovery. It would, for example, be quite wrong for a counsellor to agree, openly or tacitly, that everything in life is as hopeless and bleak as it can often appear during the early stages of grief. This would only confirm bereaved people in their despair. The idea that there is a pathway through grief, that it is possible to recover, whilst it cannot be imposed on the bereaved person, should always be retained by the counsellor, and offered in reassurance to grieving people.

Anger

Anger is a common reaction to loss, and a normal element in the process of recovery. It has a long history: Kübler-Ross (1970) describes American Indian cultures which talked of evil spirits, and shot arrows into the air to drive the spirits away. Anger fulfils this purpose too, with spears and arrows often replaced by fists, words and even lawsuits.

Anger arises when the reality of loss can no longer be denied, and bereaved people begin to experience the full pain and finality of their loss. The anger that follows is often irrational and uncontrolled, with the individual lashing out carelessly and abruptly at any available target. It can occur at any time after the period of initial shock, sometimes remaining latent until it erupts suddenly without apparent reason. Anger arises from a number of sources:

- the unfairness and injustice of loss
- fear of life without the deceased
- feelings of disappointment, impotence, helplessness
- a sense of abandonment
- the destruction of peace, stability and happiness.

The functional importance of anger is the relief it can bring to bereaved people. For those who feel abandoned and powerless it is an attempt to change their role from 'victim' to 'attacker'. In this sense, it can help them feel that they are reasserting some control over their life.

Anger represents an outlet for disbelief and frustration, protecting the individual from unwanted intimacy and underlying despair. Bereaved people can feel the unfairness, futility and injustice of the event, and, devoid of a convincing explanation, they seek to place blame, discover a scapegoat.

For many people, anger is alarming and can lead to considerable guilt and fear when out of character. Their anger has to be directed somewhere, and usually no-one is spared: relatives, friends, doctors, medical staff, clergy; everyone can come in for blame.

The loss was unfair or unjust

- It was unfair on the deceased, who should have been allowed more time to live, and to continue enjoying life.

- Alternatively, anger can be directed towards the deceased, who has abandoned them, left them lonely, with too many responsibilities and difficulties.

Someone is to blame

- Someone else was responsible for the loss, someone who was directly or indirectly implicated in the event, or who should have done more to prevent it.

- Alternatively, the anger can be directed inwards, the bereaved person believing that they should, or could have loved, cared or done more to prevent the loss from occurring, or used the time better. This can lead to self-abuse, or suicidal thoughts.

- Anger can be directed towards doctors, who should have acted more quickly, or tried another treatment, who should have operated, or should not have operated. No matter what anyone did, it would be wrong at such times.

- Or the anger may be directed against complete strangers, who in manifesting their happiness, perhaps quite unaware of the tragedy, appear to highlight it.

- The clergy can be targeted; they are, after all, the representatives of God who allowed this to happen.

- Ultimately, the anger can be directed at God, who, if (s)he was really caring, would not have allowed it to happen.

Significant loss can demonstrate the unfairness and futility of the world. The 'why me' question can generate resentment against anyone who appears to be happy, or anyone who has not yet faced serious loss. There are other people who should have died, either with less impact, or with greater justice.

When anger is expressed

When anger is directed against the closest, most supportive friends and relatives, often for no better reason than their immediate availability, such anger is often accepted; in grief the normal laws of inter-personal behaviour are often suspended:

> 'Even outbursts of anger, which would normally produce reciprocal aggressive behaviour, are treated with sympathy and respect.' (Parkes and Weiss, 1983)

Yet unless the meaning of such misdirected anger is understood, it is hard to accept, and can ultimately be destructive to relationships. Whilst relatives and friends expect distress and sadness, they may consider anger, personally directed, as unacceptable. Anger can exacerbate old family quarrels, or lead to the emergence of new disputes, sometimes over the reading of wills, or the ownership and inheritance of belongings.

The counsellor must pass tolerantly and non-judgementally through anger. The counsellor's skill is to recognise the protective mechanism of anger and its function. Understanding that anger directed at them 'does not belong to them' is important, enabling the recognition that the individual is coping with their distress in the only way they can at that time.

Anger should be expressed, and recognised as valid. It should be shared rather than redirected or discounted. The challenge for counsellors is not to react defensively, but to recognise it without retaliation. Unhelpful responses might include:

- 'You are being silly.'
- 'You cannot possibly believe that.'
- 'You cannot continue behaving like this.'

It is important to be direct and straightforward, recognising distressed people's feelings, trying to understand the meaning of their behaviour, and encouraging them to express their anger:

- 'Perhaps I cannot help bring him back; but maybe you can tell me more calmly how you are going to feel without him.'
- 'I cannot possibly know how you feel; but I would be interested to hear if you want to tell me.'
- 'I recognise that you feel that what has happened is unfair and unreasonably, and I would like to know how this makes you feel?'
- 'I know that you are angry now and that you do not want to talk; but when you want to, I will be happy to listen to you.'

When anger is repressed

Other people are unable or unwilling to experience and express anger openly. Many older people have learnt that anger and hate are unacceptable feelings, too frightening to harbour, or inappropriate for mourning; so they must be avoided or denied. Any inadvertent expression of anger can lead to strong feelings of guilt, so they cut their feelings off, and adopt other protective emotions, such as despair and hopelessness to express their distress. These 'protective' patterns can replace anger, but are often damaging, and prevent progress towards recovery. Depression has been described as

anger turned inward onto one's self

instead of outwardly towards others. Many people seek to control their anger, and deny its existence. Often, people feel more comfortable being depressed than angry – it usually generates more sympathy.

The ability of the counsellor to sense underlying feelings of anger, and to encourage its expression as representing their deep pain is important. When faced with anger, a counsellor should aim to:

- recognise, tolerate and understand the feelings underlying the anger
- help the individual gradually to recognise, express and accept anger and resentment rather than allowing them to result in guilt and depression

- help others who may be hurt or confused, to understand that anger is natural, not personally directed, and related to frustration and power-lessness
- help the individual understand that it is difficult for others to be tolerant of their anger.

Some people need encouragement to express and acknowledge their anger verbally, for when anger remains unexpressed it makes peace of mind impossible, often leading to outbreaks of physical violence, or unreasonable resentment which can jeopardise relationships with family and friends at a vulnerable time.

The expression of anger can help the individual feel safe enough to recognise and accept their feelings, trusting that the counsellor will not be overwhelmed by it, and that they too can eventually manage the feeling.

The counsellor can help bereaved people understand that anger stems from the intense pain of loss. But it can be counter-productive to approach the issue of anger directly, for example, by asking if the anger arises from their bereavement. Most people will either deny it, or fail to recognise the connection. It is usually better to deal with anger indirectly, through talking about loss, and giving people an opportunity to talk about some of their more negative feelings. As Worden (1982) says, it is important to help people find a better balance between their negative and positive feelings. Negative feelings are a way of avoiding sadness and admitting their loss.

Yet whilst anger can be an important part of the recovery process, and can be accepted for a time, if it continues too long it can indicate an expenditure of energy in an unhelpful direction. It is important that anger is time-limited, and that bereaved people come to terms with the cause of their anger.

Certainly, anger is not a solution. Staudacher (1988) suggests two questions to determine whether anger is helpful:

- Is anger providing temporary energy, or depleting what small amount of energy the individual has?
- Is the anger being used by the individual, or is it using the individual?

If the answers indicate that the anger is draining, consuming, or manipulating the individual, professional help may be required.

Fear and anxiety

Fear is a common element in the bereavement process. It can arise from the prospect of facing the world diminished or alone, by separation from a person who has been an important part of their personal identity for many years. Sometimes, anxiety and fear alternate with shock and numbness, with fear arising when the individual can no longer remember what the deceased looked like, or they feel they cannot cope with life alone:

- the fear of being alone in a house that now seems cold and empty
- the fear that other close friends might die, or desert us
- the fear of illness or injury, particularly if this was the cause of death.

Loss and separation produce feelings of insecurity, demonstrating how little control we have over events and circumstances. For older people it can seem to overthrow stable forms of social functioning that have endured for many years, shattering previously secure patterns of life. People feel lost when they face a future that is at best unclear, and at worst frightening in its uncertainty. For many people this can lead to an estrangement from life and its new realities, and the belief that life has become unsafe, a dangerous situation in which they have lost confidence.

Anxiety arises from feelings of helplessness and uncertainty about the new situation, separated from a major source of support, comfort and reassurance. Older people can be uncertain about how they will manage, and doubts can torment and overwhelm an already anxious mind. Anxiety increases in proportion with the degree of dependence. Often bereaved people have to manage alone, undertaking tasks they have not done for many years.

Anxiety can also cause the return of many, former irrational fears, perhaps concerning the dark, sleeping alone, footsteps, or living in an empty house. Former childhood fears can return, leading to regressive behaviour which for many older people can lead to bewilderment, shame, alarm and despondency, and a feeling that they have little control over their behaviour, and fears of mental breakdown.

Anxiety, particularly in older age, can also relate to a heightened awareness of personal mortality, often intensified following the death of someone close. Anxiety can also produce a number of physical symptoms, such as:

- a dry mouth
- constricted throat and chest
- breathing difficulties
- heaviness in the stomach.

- heart palpitations
- restlessness
- loss of energy

These symptoms can exacerbate this state of uncertainty. Some older people will welcome and benefit from discussion about personal mortality and death. Others will be more reluctant. For those who are worried about their health, a medical examination can be helpful.

Inability to cope with anxiety and fear can be a major reason for failure to recover from bereavement. If older people believe that the future offers few prospects other than pain, loneliness, hardship and other problems and difficulties, it is unlikely that they will be able to redirect their energy towards creating a new future.

Anxiety usually eases with time and the realisation that people can, in fact, manage. Counselling enables people to share their fears and anxieties, and place them into a wider perspective. The counsellor's initial response to anxiety and fear should be to assure them that nothing needs to be done at present, beyond relaxation, rest and making sense of what has happened to them.

As time passes, the counsellor can begin to examine what lies behind the fears and anxieties, which aspects of future life hold the most fears, and which produce most anxiety. These can lay in many areas, the most important being:

● financial management
● household management
● making new friends.

The counsellor can help people recognise the ways they managed before loss, thereby helping to place their problems into perspective. Then, small tasks or goals can be set, aimed to assist individuals to work in the areas where their fears and anxieties exist, thereby developing their skills, confidence, motivation and self-esteem. If these small tasks are successfully achieved, more difficult tasks can be set, and new challenges can be taken up.

Where the problem is a lack of knowledge or skill, people can be brought in to assist in developing an individual's ability to cope in those areas. Often, older people will welcome a new challenge, perhaps in an area in which they have never been allowed or required to develop an interest.

Guilt and remorse

Guilt is also a normal feature of bereavement. People can often feel completely debilitated by guilt, believing that for some reason they have done something wrong, committed some important error, for which they have been punished by their loss. Most guilt may be entirely unfounded and irrational, although the feelings it generates are no less real.

One purpose of guilt is to deny the reality of death, a method of keeping the deceased person alive, at least in the mind, and refusing to move on towards recovery. The outcome of unresolved or unforgiven guilt is often a distressing anxiety with which people feel unable to cope.

Guilt often arises from the desire, increasing in the modern world, to be in control of events, to feel that life should be more ordered than it is, or indeed, can be. There is a growing belief in an age which believes that science, and man's ability to control life, is all-powerful, that life should constitute an ordered existence. When this proves untenable, then it must be someone's responsibility.

Often, the people held responsible are ourselves. If we had taken some action the loss might not have happened. Self-reproach is often a feature of bereavement when there has been little pre-warning (Parkes and Weiss, 1983), even when such reasoning is quite unjustified.

There are, in fact, many reasons for feelings of guilt; in the absence of an acceptable reason for loss, people can easily feel that they were at fault, have not loved or cared enough, been disloyal, or contributed in some thought or action to bringing about death. Guilt is usually irrational; it can arise from any event, thought, feeling, or memory, the sins of both commission and omission, all of which the counsellor needs to understand:

- some feel guilty that they are not experiencing what they believe to be the 'correct' level of pain and sadness
- some feel that everything that might have been done was not done: better medical care should have been provided; the doctor should have come sooner; the operation should have been allowed, (or not, as the case may be)
- guilt can arise from failing to be present when death occurred, missing the chance to say 'goodbye', of easing the pain or loneliness of death; some people feel that had they been present they could have prevented death occurring
- guilt can arise from having felt 'good' about the loss: perhaps after a long illness, carers may have wished for some respite from pain and suffering, or felt relief from death
- guilt can arise from real or assumed shortcomings within a relationship; a sense of personal failure, unfinished business, regrets based on 'I should have ...' and 'if only ... ' thoughts
- guilt can arise from angry statements, harsh words or thoughts, which were never withdrawn or rectified before death
- 'survivor guilt' can arise from confused feelings of anger, relief or regret after surviving an accident; the guilt of being left alive; why they, and not the deceased has survived
- some feel guilty when life after bereavement is easier; perhaps the deceased had required major care; or money, property or possessions, were inherited
- there is the cultural idea that death is selective, that God, or Fate should have chosen 'us' rather than 'them'; the idea that death and survival can be traded, that one life can be exchanged or substituted for another.

All these situations can lead to guilt, remorse and self-recrimination. Older people can be particularly prone to feeling that they, rather than anyone else, should have been taken, pointing to their advanced years, ill-health, their perceived lack of importance or value, to suggest that the life of the deceased should have been spared, and they should have died instead.

The consequences of guilt can be devastating. It can lead to excessive sadness, despair, disillusionment with life, and both physical and mental illness. Such torment can persist for several months, with the individual becoming obsessive about the circumstances surrounding the death. The remorse arising from guilt becomes more unbearable when it is too late to rectify the omission, or to gain forgiveness.

Although most guilt is irrational and unrealistic, the counselling task should not dismiss such feelings, if only in the interests of maintaining 'unconditional positive regard'. Too often, people struggling with guilt are told that they are:

'being silly'

or told not to

'carry on like that'

or reassured that they should not blame themselves. Such reaction is usually meant to offer comfort and consolation, but the effect is often to deny that the person's feelings of guilt are real. It is also important to realise that people who feel guilty tend to dislike sympathy and reassurance if they feel that they do not deserve kindness of any sort.

Some guilt may be appropriate and justified; an individual may have contributed to their loss, perhaps when they have hurt someone they loved, and they can no longer repair or heal the hurt. There are few perfect relationships, ambivalent feelings of love and hate can exist side-by-side, and some attempt to distinguish between what is real and unreal guilt is often necessary.

Initially, counsellors should accept what is said, perhaps questioning general superstitions or fallacies, but neither denying the wrong people believe they have done, nor apportioning blame. To reveal guilty feelings is a sign of trust and acceptance, and the counsellor should always approach people's feelings sensitively, and, only in time, to assess their personal role in the loss.

Yet, it is also important to realise that people who feel guilty choose to do so. Guilt is a self-selected behaviour. People who feel guilty following loss usually do so because they wish to feel guilty, not because there is any rational reason for doing so. There are three 'self-flagellating' advantages arising from guilt, all encouraging the maintenance of guilty feelings:

- guilt represents the self-infliction of pain at a time when grief makes this easier than to accept that loss is a normal life-experience; guilt may be easier, or more acceptable than recommencing life
- self-blame removes responsibility from other people, supporting and underlining personal feelings of inadequacy, and confirming low self-image
- the expression of personal guilt emphasises personal distress; its reward is increased sympathy, and procuring of continued support.

Unresolved guilt delays personal recovery, and undermines self-confidence. The problem with guilt is that it is an obstructive, paralysing emotion in which it is easy to become permanently locked. Many people cannot bring themselves to talk about their guilt, too ashamed to admit such feelings to anyone. For some people the burden of guilt becomes so great that it never emerges into full consciousness. Instead there is an unconscious attempt to compensate, perhaps through an over-expensive funeral, or idealising the deceased. This can mean that powerfully destructive feelings, often totally irrational, are difficult to challenge and overcome.

But guilt does have to be challenged. All three reasons for continuing guilt need to be discussed, and, where necessary, the foundations upon which personal guilt is based challenged. To do otherwise would merely confirm people in their guilt, and the personal distress that arises from it. Counselling can help because the irrationality of guilt renders itself to 'reality testing'. Thus, if an individual states:

'I did not do enough,'

it leads to the questions:

'What did you do?'
'What else could you have done?'

At the end of such a process, bereaved people can be helped to realise that perhaps there was nothing more that they could have done. Guilt is usually short-lived, and, once recognised, the feelings begin to wane, and recovery can commence.

Crying and tears

Crying is a natural reaction to grief. Tears can help people express, and release their pain. Yet often, there is strong pressure to avoid crying, based on social discomfort and the perceived need to 'protect' people from the uneasiness often felt in the company of tears. This is often based on the misguided, but dominant idea of 'being strong', particularly with men. It is important to recognise that crying fulfils several functions:

- it is a sign of emotional distress
- it may seek to call back, or be reunited with the deceased
- it can be a device to solicit a sympathetic or protective response from other people.

The time-honoured observation that tears have potential healing value in relieving emotional stress may be in the process of being scientifically confirmed. Stress is known to cause a chemical imbalance in the body, and some research suggests that tears can helpfully remove toxic substances from the body at such times. The chemical content of 'emotional' tears is known to be different from tears secreted by eye irritation.

Crying is difficult for many people. There are many devices used to prevent crying which are not only inappropriate, but unhelpful when dealing with grief. Some people will suppress their tears in front of friends. Others fear that crying is undignified, or embarrassing to other people, and might strain relationships. The phrase 'to break down' indicates that weeping is something to be avoided.

Counselling should encourage the process of crying, for it can provide a release mechanism for grief. It is certainly important for people to know that their crying will not cause you to leave, and some useful phrases or comments might be:

- 'Please feel that you can cry; perhaps you should.'
- 'It must be hard to feel so unhappy and not to cry.'
- 'Crying may help; it is unnecessary to hold your tears back.'
- 'It is OK to cry, I would be concerned if you did not shed a few tears.'

However, it should be realised that merely to elicit crying is insufficient. Bereaved people need to be able to identify the cause of their tears, and come to terms with it.

Unhappiness, sadness and despair

When people emerge from the early stages of grief they enter a time of acute pain and deep distress. Feelings which were previously denied have to be faced. It can be a time when the slightest reminder of loss can lead to overwhelming sadness and despair.

Despair is common: despair at what is lost and the apparent emptiness of their lives. Waves of unhappiness can arise, often accompanied by intense crying, outbursts of anger, feelings of guilt, and periods of bewilderment. The prospect of a life alone can seem unbearable, and totally consuming. Concern focuses on the deceased; there is little time or energy for anything else; other activity can seem to be entirely without purpose. There is often little investment in the present, and often none at all in the future.

There are many physical symptoms, and stress-induced illnesses which can arise from such sorrow:

- headaches
- aches and pains
- tiredness
- nightmares
- heart palpitations
- appetite loss
- weight loss
- sleeplessness.

If the individual can sleep, it can be a temporary release which many will want extend for as long as possible, perhaps spending the greater part of the day dozing.

It is widely agreed that a failure to experience, or the repression of, unhappiness and sadness, a significant part of any normal grief reaction, can delay the process of recovery. Over the last century, psychoanalysis has indicated that those who repress an outward show of grief are likely to suffer in other ways, including physical and mental illness. The more people are able to feel, and come to terms with their emotions, the more possible it becomes to pass successfully through the bereavement process.

Counselling can be helpful in achieving this as it enables the individual to express their pain. The counsellor should try to empathise with the individual, and look at the situation from his/her point of view. They should be allowed to be sad, and free from requests to 'cheer up', or to stop 'being morbid', or in any other way made to feel that their sadness is upsetting other people. The simple acknowledgement that another person is interested in how they feel can confirm a person's sense of identity and self-esteem.

The counsellor should ask questions and seek clarification, since this encourages an understanding that their feelings are considered important. If the individual can be encouraged to believe that they will not lose control, or become totally depressed if they acknowledge their feelings, they can begin to acknowledge the reality and meaning of loss.

The counsellor should also seek to discern the individual's understanding of the process of grieving. The knowledge that grief will not last forever may not reduce current pain, but can be helpful in enabling the individual to endure it. Bereaved people need to be assured of:

- the transient nature of grief
- that distress levels will decline
- that they can recover in time.

Often people can be helped by recalling previous periods of grief, how they felt at the time, and how they recovered. Older people often have an advantage in being able to call upon their experience. When they realise that they have grieved before and recovered, and that grief does not last forever, they can begin to accept that they can recover again.

This can lead to a discussion about the skills and attitudes which allowed them to recover previously, and which they still retain for use in the current situation, including perhaps their:

- sense of perspective
- resilience
- endurance
- courage
- capacity to distance
- sense of humour.
- patience
- perseverance

Helplessness and hopelessness

In the midst of sadness, feelings of helplessness and hopelessness have particular meaning for older people. Many can feel this in relation to the ageing process generally. When significant loss becomes an additional burden, the ability to remain optimistic, useful and hopeful diminishes still further. Often a sense of hopelessness about the prospect of re-establishing a worthwhile quality of life develops.

An individual's life history, personal characteristics, and capacity for optimism and resilience, can determine how well an older person is able to cope with major loss. Yet even the most resilient person, faced with a combination of increasing age and major bereavement, may feel that they are no longer able to make any worthwhile impression on their personal circumstances.

These feelings and attitudes towards life can appear intractable, and deeply depressing. Most people who face significant loss will feel helpless; but those who have lost a highly dependent relationship may feel completely overwhelmed by the problems of future life. It then becomes exceedingly difficult to have any impact upon the way they feel, dominated as they are by low self-image.

Spending time with them, listening, encouraging them to undertake small tasks, reminiscence, seeking the involvement of friends and relations (particularly those who have survived similar bereavement, and experienced similar feelings), trying to look optimistically on the events and situations that occur, are all techniques that can help. Perseverance is vital for it has to be recognised that moving through strong feelings of helplessness and hopelessness may be a lengthy, emotionally difficult process.

Hopelessness about the future can mean that people continue to live in the past. Many bereaved people choose to maintain feelings that immobilise and depress them, believing that such feelings will never subside, and perhaps not wanting them to as this is how they can maintain their link with the deceased.

It is often counter-productive to encourage positive thinking in such circumstances. The best response to expressions of hopelessness and helplessness is to agree that this is how they feel currently, but to suggest that they might not always feel this way.

Yearning

Yearning is the painful experience of intense longing for reunion, and the feelings of aloneness and sadness that accompany this. The process of moving towards recovery without the deceased can seem unthinkable, even disloyal. The yearning mind is constantly balancing the reality that the dead person will never return with the desire for reunion. Often, this involves constant repetition of the same thoughts and ideas to the extent that yearning will often absorb their entire energy and interest.

Yearning indicates that bereaved people are beginning to realise, however reluctantly, that the deceased can no longer be part of their lives, a slow but painful recognition that they will have to separate themselves, although they may still want to avoid having to do so.

Yearning has to be experienced as part of the recovery process. Reminiscence is one way of dealing with yearning, as it can provide the opportunity of discussing feelings about loss whilst at the same time emphasising that loss is the reality. People who yearn for reunion will usually relish the opportunity to reminisce, but carers can be discouraged because of the apparent desire of bereaved people to talk endlessly and repetitively about their memories. This can be irritating, yet the process provides the counsellor with an opportunity, so often missed, to allow bereaved people to express themselves. Reliving and remembering is a helpful activity for several reasons:

- it provides a safety valve for feelings that may need to be expressed
- it can help clarify confused feelings and thoughts
- it can reawaken important memories that indicate that the dead person can never be entirely lost within their memory
- it can help place memories in the past, and place them in the context of the present and future.

With care and time, yearning will subside, although some people are reluctant to relinquish it as they feel that this implies that their commitment to the deceased is declining. This need not be so; it means only that energies are being redirected, and that the individual is recovering by allowing other people, other situations, and other priorities to begin to reduce the amount of time for yearning.

Yet, the degree of yearning and sadness is considered an important early indicator of a recovery process that may go wrong (Clayton *et al.*, 1969; Parkes and Weiss, 1983), with the intensity of grief at the time of bereavement being directly related to poor outcome. This means that counsellors who confine their activity to eliciting expressions of grief could be in danger of confirming unhappiness, and colluding with the perpetuation of chronic grief.

Self-neglect

One consequence of bereavement in older age, arising from guilt, anxiety and low self-esteem, is self-neglect. This can take many forms, including failure to:

- eat properly
- maintain standards of hygiene
- maintain social engagement.

Like guilt, self-neglect is often a form of self-punishment, bringing with it all the 'advantages' that this can offer lonely and depressed people.

There is a widespread belief that self-neglect is a necessary part of grief, a way of indicating our hurt, and how painful our bereavement experience has been. Self-neglect is undertaken as penance for whatever blame people feel should be attached to them.

Self neglect needs to be challenged gently and kindly, while leaving the individual in little doubt that self-neglect is unhelpful, and that such behaviour will, not by itself, elicit concern and support. As Tatelbaum (1981) says:

> 'In many cases it takes a life crisis, such as a loss or a move, for us to recognize our need for our own love, concern, and support. As important as it is for us to take care of ourselves every day, our need for self-support and self-concern is critical when we are grieving. If we neglect ourselves at such times, we impede our recovery.'

Counselling can help people recognise the importance of self-love and self-care. It can focus on personal interests and values. It can explore the activities that would be of interest, and give pleasure to the individual. It can encourage the individual to take up such activities in the interests of their own self-esteem, on the basis that by accepting personal needs, regardless of what they are, we can make life more enjoyable and rewarding.

Counselling can help acknowledge that self-neglect is not a true reflection either of love or faithfulness for the deceased, that no-one, alive or dead, would want to see the person they have loved suffer in such a way, and in their name.

Activity is the key to self-care. Tatelbaum (1981) suggests that the starting point might be to encourage the creation of a 'memorial' to the lost person. Perhaps this can be done in response to questions which enquire:

> 'How/why was she/he special?'

and

> 'What can be done to remember him/her?'

These questions are also helpful in focusing thoughts about the deceased in the reality of the present, rather than in the unobtainable past. Counselling can then encourage people to pay more attention to personal needs by encouraging other enjoyable pursuits; perhaps spending time shopping, reading, taking a bath, or an afternoon sleep; or travelling to places of interest.

The specific activity is unimportant, and will arise from individual interests. What is important is that the activity responds to personal needs, interests and pleasures.

Depression

Bereavement and depression are inextricably linked. Collick (1982) describes depression as a time of dejection, poverty of spirit, an overwhelming grey bleakness and hopeless despair. It is a time when apathy dominates. Depressed people usually refuse to use their initiative, relinquish self-reliance, and lose self-esteem and self-respect. Activity is undertaken without enthusiasm, often with strong expressions of self-pity; depressed people eat without enjoyment, sleep without rest; and display a resigned disinterest in their pain, and their future.

Yet care needs to be taken when using the term 'depression' because of its close association with mental illness. Medically, 'depression' denotes mental illness; but the word is often used more 'loosely' to describe feelings which are similar to, but more than unhappiness, sadness and despair. The problem is that when profound sadness is labelled 'depression', it may lead to people receiving medical treatment for a condition that is a common companion to the normal process of bereavement.

Depression, in its looser sense, represents an unwillingness to remain engaged in social activity. Depression can protect people from feelings of unbearable anger and hate by cutting off feeling altogether. It is the antithesis of feeling: the individual no longer wishes to experience the intensity of yearning and loss. It often manifests itself in the form of total blankness.

Such 'lack of feeling' may be wrongly interpreted by carers; depression remains a time of intense pain, often entwined with periods of detachment and lack of emotion. A depressed state has many features:

- irritability
- pessimism
- hopelessness
- loss of appetite
- restlessness
- self-blame
- social withdrawal
- emptiness
- powerlessness
- lack of concentration
- lack of confidence
- loss of sexual drive
- apathy
- lethargy
- despair
- tearfulness
- tiredness
- insomnia.

Yet depression indicates a subtle change in focus. Instead of being preoccupied with the deceased, depressed people tend to become preoccupied with themselves, perhaps more involved in self-doubt, self-blame, or self-persecution. Yet it is a significant change as it means that attention is moving away from the past towards the present; to life as it is as opposed to life as it was.

Thus, paradoxically, depression occurs when mourning is moving towards recovery, so it can be an encouraging sign, even if a difficult, undesirable one for carers. It is a period of painful despair, but rather than denying what has happened, it also involves a conscious process of relinquishing, or 'giving up'.

It is the misery of grief, and the emptiness of depression that eventually permits recovery; the pain demands relief. This is not done by forgetting the past, but by accepting that the past cannot be recovered. Depression can be a mobilising force, encouraging more outgoing, adventurous behaviour which can allow older people to discover facets of themselves long forgotten, or never before tested.

Depression is a passive rather than an active state. It requires less effort to be resigned to reality than to fight against it. The emotional energy demanded by anger and yearning is too great to continue indefinitely; depression represents the time when people decide to struggle no more. Moods of depression and yearning can often alternate. The intense feeling and severe emotional disturbance associated with yearning may decline gradually into depression, and then suddenly the painful emotions of loss may return again to overwhelm the individual.

Many typical responses to depression are unhelpful:

- 'Pull yourself together.'
- 'Snap out of it.'
- 'Stop wallowing in self-pity.'

All discount the purpose of depression, which is a refusal to act and to feel because to do so has become too painful. Many depressed people, when counselled sympathetically, will admit that they no longer wish to continue living. Relatively few bereaved people seriously contemplate suicide, but it would be wrong to ignore the possibility that someone might consider ending their lives. It is always correct to consider making a referral to the doctor, to trained psychiatric help, or even to the Samaritans.

Working with depression requires patience, and where it persists counsellors will require support. Counselling provides depressed people with a listening ear, and time to consider the future. This becomes important when depression leads to social withdrawal, for this completes a damaging circularity:

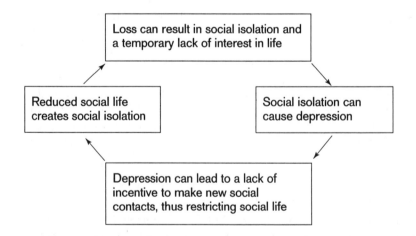

With older people this can be a damaging sequence which, far from leading to recovery from bereavement, returns them to back towards hopelessness and despair.

The initial counselling task is to set recovery as the essential goal, encouraging the individual to live each day as it comes, dealing with the regular routine of living, and the decisions that have to be made, as and when they arise. The time when people can look to the future and see something worthwhile may still be some time ahead. The path to recovery requires sufficient perspective to understand which part of the journey can be accomplished that day, whilst at the same time maintaining sight of the eventual destination.

It is common for depressed people to be resistant to accepting their underlying feelings. It may be necessary to comment on this:

- 'Whenever I suggest that you may feel (sad) (unhappy) (angry) you seem unable to respond. Why do you think this is?'
- 'Whenever I mention (your loss) you do not show any reaction; it is as if you did not know, or dare not talk about what has happened.'

Depression represents a loss of hope, so it is important for carers to hold on to their sense of hope, whilst not denying their feelings of hopelessness. If carers of older people lose hope, a sense of what might be possible in future, further contact and support might become mutually depressing:

- 'You seem to be in such despair you can see no way out of your situation. I wonder if you can help me understand your melancholy, because I can see you doing so much with the rest of your life if you only wanted to do so.'

Ultimately, depression, although it might protect the person from less tolerable feelings of guilt and helplessness, is also an intolerable experience. Eventually, other people find it uncomfortable, leading to further isolation and loneliness, and ultimately, to suicidal thoughts.

Depression that continues over a long period, and which comes to dominate a person's entire life is known as 'endogenous' depression, signifying a depression that exists deep within the individual. This is not the depression normally caused by temporary 'external' factors such as bereavement, but is usually embedded in the personality. It is also important to understand that depression can lead to mental illness, particularly if the individual is left unsupported. Carers need to seek advice when depression is 'stuck' and a referral to a doctor for specialist help is necessary.

Bereavement as mental illness

Grief can exacerbate psychiatric illness, particularly following the loss of a major relationship. Throughout the mourning process, bereaved people will experience feelings they know to be irrational, but over which they seem to have little control. They may feel confused, unable to order their thoughts, and have difficulty in concentrating. This can manifest itself in behaviour which people consider to be entirely contrary to their normal personality and character, and can include:

- irrational fears and thoughts

- an inability to concentrate on important tasks
- an inability to think clearly or sensibly
- making strange statements or remarks
- unusual behaviour which the individual is unable to control
- strange thoughts and imaginings.

The experience of visual and auditory hallucinations can be particularly frightening, with their close association with mental instability. Many bereaved people report having visions of the dead person, and life-like dreams which can be disturbing and confusing. In such circumstances, people fear that they may be going mad, particularly older people who may associate them with signs of early senile dementia.

Again, such symptoms are normal for people suffering significant loss, and they are usually transient phenomena, generally not extending longer than a few weeks into the mourning process. They result from the upheaval caused by significant loss and should not be considered a sign of early mental illness. The counsellor, in offering a listening ear, and responding with caring and understanding to expressions of anxiety, can help to ensure that the 'normal' does not transform itself into the 'abnormal' – mental illness.

These feelings can be very strong, and their impact on behaviour so distinct they can lead to diagnoses of mental illness or dementia. The danger of labelling is considerable. It has been estimated that up 15 per cent of people with psychological conditions who pass through the mental health clinics in Massachusetts had suffered some unresolved grief reaction (Lazare, 1979). Bowlby (1980) confirmed this clinical experience, stating that much psychiatric illness, including anxiety states, depressive illness, hysteria, and some character disorders, can be an expression of pathological mourning.

Yet the worry caused to people who may feel that they are losing control of their minds may itself be sufficient to begin the process of mental breakdown, and this needs to be recognised as a possible risk when grieving is very intense. Again, when this seems to be the case, a referral to a doctor may be appropriate.

Recognising emotional acceptance

The ability of bereaved people to accept loss emotionally is not age related; older people are quite able to restore their interest and involvement in life. If the motivation and desire to do so are present it will happen regardless of age; if they are not, younger people are equally unlikely to reinvest in the rest of their lives.

Parkes and Weiss (1983) felt that emotional acceptance took place when bereaved people no longer felt the need to avoid reminders of loss for fear of being flooded by grief, pain or remorse. They indicated that to reach acceptance there had to be repeated confrontation with every element of the loss until the intensity of distress was diminished to the point where it became tolerable, and the pleasure of recollection began to outweigh the pain.

Acceptance of loss does not mean that the past is forgotten. It is impossible for bereaved people to forget entirely; loss remains part of our lives. Older people, particularly those who lose long-standing relationships, may have serious difficulties coming to terms with loss; but the pain does gradually recede. For the rest of their lives there may be moments of renewed pain and sadness, but recollection will become less intense and less frequent; the pain will no longer absorb their total attention, or reduce their ability to function normally within the social setting. Intellectual and emotional acceptance of loss does not mean that life will remain unchanged; but it does mean that it can continue.

Task three: adjusting to loss

The transition from the most disabling stages of grief to an acceptance of loss does not happen quickly or painlessly, or indeed forever. Gradually, bereaved people can regain a sense of emotional sanity, personal reintegration, and social purpose. Adjusting to loss can happen when the individual is able to encompass the following:

- **The present:**
  The individual feels able to:
     cope with it
     enjoy it
     move on from it.

- **The future:**
  The individual is able to look at it with some:
     optimism
     hope
     expectation.

- **The past:**
  The individual is able to view it as:
     a place where pleasant memories exist
     a time to value and remember
     something that should not obstruct living.

Yet even when loss has been accepted, intellectually and emotionally, the practical social consequences remain. Decisions about making life adjustments become important only after people have learnt to face the new realities of life, and come to terms with the pain and significance of loss. It is only when:

- the desire for reunion is no longer seriously considered
- the duration and intensity of periods of sorrow have significantly decreased
- depression and guilt have gradually eased.

that the task of adjusting to a new environment will begin. Acceptance enables people to face the task of reinvesting in living again, and all that this implies.

This will call upon many personal strengths. Loss will force people to re-evaluate their lives and question many previous attitudes and values. It may lead to some significant changes which will now have to be considered.

Making sense of bereavement

For effective recovery people must feel that the changed world makes sense. The ability to make sense of bereavement is vital to recovery. Loss may appear unfair and irrational, the event inexplicable, meaningless, and indiscriminate. This can remain so for many years. People need to be able to understand their loss in a wider context. Any explanation of what has taken place must be felt to be true by the individual, and must answer the many 'why?' questions that loss produces. Developing such an account is a necessary although not a sufficient prerequisite for recovery.

After death, bereaved people are confronted with the meaning of life, one of the biggest mysteries mankind has battled with through the ages. Religious belief seeks to provide absolute answers to such questions, usually quite unsatisfactorily: even people with strong religious belief question them when confronted with unacceptable loss. Staudacher (1988) believes that people's beliefs about the meaning of death adopt one of following orientations:

- death is being with God in heaven
- death is an invisible force that takes you when it is your time to go
- death is a time of judgement during which your life is evaluated, with subsequent consignment to either heaven or hell
- death is non-living, the ultimate existential experience
- death is an elevation to another life, a continued existence in a realm without the consequences of human frailty, hostility, materialist values, etc.
- death is a rebirth, beginning again in a new and different life
- death is the state between two other states, as sleep is the state between two waking states.

These ideas are often too facile, too spontaneous, too glib to be excepted as stated. Many bereaved people will want to examine and discuss such ideas closely in relation to their experience, re-examining many former beliefs, and reach their own conclusions.

The reorganisation and reassessment of life

Reorganisation and reassessment can happen when the deceased is no longer the primary focus. It is often a time when bereaved people need less care, when they want to be left alone, quieter, when they begin to make small steps towards a more active social life, or start looking to engage in more fulfilling activity. The individual will begin to function more normally again:

- appetite returns
- sleep becomes easier
- energy is more readily available
- more interest is taken in life generally.

The bereavement experience often brings with it a heightened awareness of personal mortality, and the inevitable death that awaits everyone. This can lead to an opportunity to reassess ideas about the meaning of life, and to re-evaluate personal attitudes, behaviour, values and goals. Often, this can lead to an increased understanding of personal limitations, as well as opening up new possibilities.

The acceptance of loss means that the individual relinquishes many former bonds, rituals and processes that are no longer relevant. Bereaved people are often unaware of the tasks and responsibilities previously undertaken by their lost partner. These tasks will leave gaps, large and small, which will serve as a daily reminder of loss:

- the house will be empty, devoid of a former companion
- household bills require payment, and provisions have to be purchased
- meals need to be prepared
- the garden requires attention
- the bed will seem empty and cold; a sexual partner is missing
- the day needs to be passed amidst feelings of isolation and loneliness.

It can take many weeks for bereaved people to realise the full implications of loss. Many will decide that they must fulfil unaccustomed roles, see them as a challenge, and develop the new skills required. Others will be more reluctant, whilst some will do little apart from promoting their helplessness.

This adjustment is not easy and counselling can assist in answering a variety of practical questions:

- What has been lost, and what cannot now be achieved?

- What needs to be done, what are the gaps, how are they to be filled?
- What are the choices and decisions to be made?
- Who is to undertake the task?
- What are the options available?

Loneliness

Accepting the loss of significant relationships is likely to lead to feelings of loneliness. Personal relationships give meaning to life, and their loss means the forfeit of an important part of self-identity, affecting the way people feel about who they are, and what they are capable of doing.

This is particularly true for older people, who may have lost many long-standing friends within their age-group, and can be particularly vulnerable to isolation. There are often other factors which make socialising difficult, including financial stringency, feeling unsafe and vulnerable, illness, and physical disabilities, all making socialisation, visiting people, and joining groups difficult. There are several forms of loneliness (Collick, 1982):

- **Physical isolation:**
  This arises from the absence of an important person, leading to isolation, emptiness, and lack of companionship. Within the home former tasks are no longer necessary, and others which have to be undertaken only highlight the sense of loss, and the feelings of loneliness.
- **Social loneliness:**
  This arises when there is no one to go out with, to cook for, or to please. Walks and meals become solitary, and so less valuable. Holidays are either not taken, or they lose their former meaning and excitement.
- **Personal loneliness:**
  Collick (1982) believes that the most bitter loneliness comes from the loss of shared experience following bereavement. There is now only 'me' and 'mine' where once there was 'us' and 'ours'. The importance of sharing simple experiences, resolving problems and difficulties together, are all aspects of a relationship which are often taken for granted until eventually lost.

It is important to distinguish between loneliness that results from ageing within an ageist society, and loneliness brought about by bereavement. Loneliness can result from the mourning process, and is not age-related; such lonliness can come from:

- the distancing function of numbness
- the futility of searching
- the alienating effects of anger
- the humiliation of guilt
- the unattractiveness of depression.

Conversely, loneliness can arise from social structures, attitudes and expectations, which can impose enormous burdens on older people. Given their age, and ageist attitudes, bereavement can seem to constitute not a temporary loss, but a permanent, irreplaceable one. Many older bereaved people can see only bleak years in front of them; the opportunities for developing new activities and friendships seem remote. This is often made worse by the stigma of widow(er)hood, which can erect barriers to social reintegration for those who have lost important partners.

There are, however, two situations which make loneliness a particularly difficult situation to tackle:

1. Loneliness which has been experienced over a long time, often mixed with depression and self-pity, can become self-propagating. The more lonely, unhappy, depressed and unfulfilled an individual feels, the more other people are driven away. If such situations drift, loneliness can become a deeply embedded life-expectation, with hope and optimism for the future destroyed.
2. Bereavement might have occurred at a particularly unwelcome time, making it appear especially unfair and unjust. One example is that large numbers of older people die at, or shortly after retirement age, when many couples have planned, saved, and looked forward to this as an opportunity to share increased leisure time together.

Counselling can challenge some of these ageist assumptions both within the older individual and other people. It can attempt to open up new horizons for friendship and social integration (Scrutton, 1989).

By feeling isolated and lonely people are acknowledging the significance of loss, and so providing counselling opportunities. The problem is whether this can be used to turn bereavement from what can be a fatalistic, helpless and hopeless experience into positive action to remedy the situation. There are three tasks:

- to examine personal needs and interests
- to look at the options (groups, etc.) which exist within the community
- to link these together, and encourage and facilitate involvement.

Sexual losses

Often, the most pressing, but least discussed aspects of loneliness that can arise from loss, are the sexual aspects of companionship. Sex is an instinctive need which, in so many ways, constitutes an affirmation of life itself. Yet for older people, several factors inhibit sexual activity:

- the ageist view, often internalised, that older people have no further need or interest in sexual relationships
- the social reticence, strong amongst older generations, which inhibits public discussion of sex

- the fact that many older people consider marriage a once-in-a-lifetime experience, not to be repeated
- social attitudes which often take a disparaging, satirical view of remarriage in older age
- the idea that forming another sexual relationship is unfaithful, a betrayal which can cause guilt and anxiety
- the restricted opportunities older people have for meeting with other people in social settings.

The specific problems faced by older women require special mention:

- there are usually more single older women than single older men
- older women often feel intimidated by male advances, uncertain of the intentions behind even the most innocent invitations, and aware of the common idea that widows are 'fair' game
- many older women enjoy male companionship, but feel too insecure to take the initiative in issuing social invitations, or joining male company
- some older women would like to remarry, but the opportunities are limited by social, moral and ethical restrictions.

In the early stages of loss, grief can dampen, diminish and eradicate sexual feelings. Yet in time, the desire to be wanted, the warmth and comfort that closeness with another person brings, the joy of mutual physical touch, the ability to participate in giving and receiving of pleasure and reassurance, not least in sexual intercourse, reassume their former importance.

Sexual frustration can be an intense source of anguish to older bereaved people, but the reawakening of sexual feelings can also produce feelings of guilt, anxiety, and confusion when natural needs for sexual companionship confront moral and religious beliefs, and feelings of loyalty to former partners.

For many older people the loss of a sexual relationship can be considerable, and may seem frustratingly irreparable. The extent of the loss will depend on the significance that sexual activity had in the relationship, and the degree to which social, moral, religious and familial expectations restrict freedom of action.

Counselling can play an important role in helping unravel some of these conflicting pressures, although there are many obstacles that need to be overcome:

- older people may feel unable to admit missing sexual activity, making the subject difficult to broach; many will consider sexual matters to be a personal and ethical topic for private consideration only
- the subject may be discussed euphemistically, perhaps an admission of 'missing a cuddle', or more ambiguously in terms of 'companionship'; it is through these guarded forms of expression, however, that

the issues can often be tackled
- some older people, whilst admitting that they miss the pleasure and comfort of a sexual relationship, can only envisage it within the total commitment to a relationship, and inappropriate outside marriage.

Gender differences are also important. For women, discussing sexual matters may be a greater taboo than for men, although women may be more familiar with discussing their feelings.

For men, talking about sex may be more acceptable, but probably not at a 'feeling' level; men may be more reluctant to admit sexual frustration or deprivation, and can be more reluctant to discuss such matters openly.

Masturbation is an outlet for those people left without a sexual partner, but is a practice that many older people, particularly women, will not admit or wish to discuss freely. Yet masturbation can help diminish sexual tension and frustration, although most people consider it to be an inadequate substitute. Some people find that masturbation is unhelpful, and can actually underline their loss.

Older people face two opposing views about sex in old age. McNeill Taylor (1983) has outlined how these contrasting views impinge on bereaved people. On one hand, religious (especially Christian) views have supported the idea of celibacy and chastity, even in preference to marriage. Conversely, views originating in Freudian psychology recognise that enforced chastity can lead to an unhealthy repression of natural feelings that can cause emotional distress and illness. This view has made it unfashionable for people to admit to chastity in case they are thought of as being unnaturally 'repressed', or in some way guilty of denying their natural appetites. Yet for many older people, chastity is an enforced state, about which they have little choice.

Clearly, approval and disapproval of chastity are equally misguided. In dealing with older bereaved people, a balance is required between recognising natural sexual drives, and giving respect to people who choose not to, or are unable to give sex a prominent role in their lives.

Yet the importance of sexual relations should not be discounted. Parkes and Weiss (1983) found that those who recovered from bereavement best had moved toward remarriage, and those who did remarry were most content with their lives. The capacity for social engagement, including the willingness to consider remarriage, and the maintenance of friendship and family ties, was found to be both a consequence of, and a means to further recovery.

Yet even when sexual activity does recommence, normal feelings of guilt and anxiety can play a part, with men suffering from impotence or premature ejaculation, and women finding themselves unable to respond in the way they wish, or incapable of attaining orgasm. Such problems may decline with understanding and patience, but can cause embarrassment, and sometimes an unwillingness to commence a new relationship.

The role of resolutions and affirmations

People affected by trauma often make negative resolutions about their future life. These can often take the form of

'never again'

statements which pinpoint past activities or decision of being the cause of their present pain and distress. The resolve

'I will never love again'

is particularly common amongst those who have lost a close relationship. Such resolutions, made during a vulnerable, suggestible period can be influential in the way people decide to restructure their lives. Negative, depressive resolutions are a major barrier to recovery, preventing people making the most of future opportunities.

An important prerequisite to recovery is hope – the belief that recovery is possible. Beliefs are to a large extent self-fulfilling; we act according to the our beliefs, and our thoughts are sufficiently powerful to create their own reality. People can therefore determine their own limitations, as well as their own expectations.

It is important for the counsellor to discover, examine and discuss any affirmations and resolutions, particular as many people will not be aware of what they are, as they are not usually made consciously.

Counsellors can encourage bereaved people to make positive affirmations which assist in starting the process of creating change and redirection in life. Some examples of positive affirmations are given by Tatelbaum (1981):

- I will recover.
- I have courage to go through this experience, to live alone, to face grief.
- I can grow from this adversity.
- I am strong enough to cope with life as it now is.
- I can overcome my sorrow.
- I will finish with my grief and start building a new life.
- I will share loving feelings, and have no unfinished business with loved ones.
- I intend to be patient (or persevering, honest, open understanding, or any other relevant attribute).
- I intend to live my life to the full.

Where bereaved people believe that such affirmations are not possible, the counsellor can set small tasks which can lead to increasing self-confidence on a daily or weekly basis:

- I will go out tonight.
- I will dispose of the clothes of the deceased within 1 month.

- I will repaint the kitchen.
- I will go on holiday (or take part in some other pleasurable activity).

Setting future goals is important for recovery. Simonton *et al.* (1986) recommended that goals should be concrete, specific, measurable and realistic. Setting them can have several useful outcomes. It can:

- help in reinvesting in life
- help reinforce the desire to continue living
- help reassume responsibility for living
- help rebuild self-confidence
- help in focusing energies.

Towards a new identity

Older people are used to changing their identities. Most people over 50 have terminated their identity as parents. Retired people have relinquished their identity as workers. Other losses, especially the loss of a long-standing partner, require equal, if not more difficult and bewildering changes in identity. The wife is no longer married but widowed, the husband has become a widower, and both have to develop new skills to live as single people again.

Many resist the transition, fearful of their new and uncertain identity as a single person, continuing to assume that their partner is still present. They know that they are not, but find it comforting to continue in the assumption.

Others move more quickly to a new identity. The exact timing of this adjustment is unimportant; each person should be allowed their own time to grieve. The decline of traditional mourning rituals can add to uncertainty about general social expectations. The counsellor may need to help the individual balance:

- their uncertainty
- against their ability to make the necessary adjustment

- the reawakening of their desire to recommence living
- with having 'permission', or freedom from guilt, to do so.

It is crucial that older people can see the world as a place in which they are still involved, and can make an important and satisfying personal investment. In an ageist society which assumes that real life finishes after retirement, and older age is a time when people are merely waiting for death, this can require some considerable attention.

The potential opportunities of bereavement

Acceptance of loss can lead to a return to social health, but the opportunities need to be recognised. Bereaved people, regardless of age, can initiate new relationships, and discover new roles and functions. Collick suggests that acceptance arises not so much from the passage of time but from the insistent reminders that the circumstances of daily life have changed, and that former expectations, habits, and behaviour are no longer appropriate. New life patterns and arrangements often arise from the requirements of continuing life, and it is from these that new opportunities can arise.

If there is to be hope following bereavement, loss should not be accepted as an entirely negative experience. Every loss offers an opportunity for change and adjustment. Many people, regardless of age, find that they want, or perhaps are able for the first time to change their way of life, values, and attitudes. They find that they can move in new directions, and are more able to commit themselves to causes and ideas which have previously played a less important part of their lives.

Such reassessment can profoundly change priorities, personal goals, and future social participation. Recovery offers many older people the possibility of change:

- loss can bring about major changes in personal identity
- time-honoured activities can suddenly lose their importance
- new life-perspectives, a revised set of activities, values, and friendships can be adopted
- new plans and ideas can transform the future into something more challenging and exciting.

Indeed, the more significant the loss the more opportunity for change arises. Every aspect of life is called into question and profoundly altered. Life, even in old age, has proved to be more fragile, dangerous, and unpredictable than previously assumed. What is left of life can be more deeply cherished. Remaining relationships can change after bereavement; some people move closer to their existing friends; others move away and form entirely new liaisons.

Even former beliefs can be changed. Tatelbaum (1981) suggests that this can start when people become aware that beliefs affect outcomes in our lives, and that, like habits, they are taken for granted and never re-examined. She suggests that people should write down what they believe, and then re-examine the beliefs to see if they still make sense, if they still fit into the new realities of life, to make decisions about whether they still wish to maintain them or would prefer to examine others to see if they fit their new situation more accurately.

Acceptance allows people to examine the potential of the future life, to discover new activities, interests and friends, and, through these, gradually to feel more able, more confident. Eventually, they may be able to experience contentment and fulfilment, to permit laughter and gaiety, and begin to enjoy life again; moreover, they may do so without guilt. In this way, older people can emerge from grief creatively, turning personal tragedy into an event which leads to a re-examination of what remains of life, and what they wish to do with it.

Finishing

Finishing is a concept used in Gestalt therapy, and involves facing the problem of ending relationships whether lost through death or other forms of separation (Tatelbaum, 1981). Finishing can be achieved through the 'Empty Chair' exercise, in which the individual is encouraged to express whatever feeling comes to mind, possible assisted by suggestions about how they can start. 'I ... ' sentences elicit personal feelings most successfully:

- 'I am sad.'
- 'I still miss you.'
- 'I am angry at you.'

Other useful sentences are those beginning with 'I wish ...':

- 'I wish you were still here.'
- 'I wish I could say sorry.'

Completing these simple sentences can help people express their feelings. One way to elicit deeper feelings, which may remain difficult to admit, is to encourage people to state something they know either to be untrue, or which possibly might be true. If saying it sounds 'right', then it becomes possible to continue along that path, leading to the admission of feelings previously denied.

It is also possible for a friend to answer on behalf of the deceased, or to ask the individual to guess what the lost person might have said in response to their statements.

Finishing is a method which can confirm that the grieving process has been successfully completed. The individual can be asked to state:

'I feel that I have finished with you now'

and then to try the reverse. Whichever sounds more comfortable, or natural, is probably correct.

In memoriam

Even in the most successful recovery from bereavement, personal memories of the deceased will remain important. Throughout the recovery process, and particularly as people recover from the full pain of grief, the creation of individualised 'memorials' to the deceased can be helpful, ensuring that the deceased is remembered in a positive, ongoing way, and reassuring the survivor that this can be so.

One frequent fear is that the deceased will be forgotten, or that the deceased will not be remembered distinctly enough. Bereaved people often want to retain something to commemorate a loved person to ensure this does not happen.

A memorial does not have to mean the erection of large buildings or statues; nor does it have to mean the refusal to move clothes and belongings; both have more to do with denial than recovery. There is a tradition of 'in memoria' entries in local papers; the grave is another physical reminder.

Even simpler ideas involve helping people to collect together important mementos of the deceased:

- photographs
- old letters
- paper clippings
- mementos of all descriptions.

These can be amalgamated into a scrapbook or photograph album. For people who are sufficiently motivated, material can be gathered to write a life history of the deceased, and the relationship they shared.

There is a growing trend to donate money to a church, a favourite charity, or sponsor a seat in the local park. In many cases, it is possible that the name of the deceased can be engraved, or associated in some way with the gift. Increasingly, people prefer to remember their dead with something living, perhaps by planting a shrub or tree in memory of the deceased. The Woodland Trust will do this.

Task four: social reinvestment

'Mourning has a quite precise psychical task to perform: its function is to detach the survivors' memories and hopes from the dead.'
(Freud, 1913).

Personal fulfilment is closely related to the quality of our social relationships, and the loss of an important person can be a devastating blow to morale, sometimes causing a complete breakdown of social contact. Yet there is a time to grieve and a time to recommence living. Worden's final recovery task is to redirect life towards other relationships and activities. Many bereaved people require help with their uncertainty about such reinvestment, especially if they feel that in doing so they may dishonour the memory of the deceased. Some older people may prefer to fall back on romantic notions of loyalty and 'marriage for life', and accept that they will lead their lives in increasing loneliness. Yet the formation of new personal relationships can be vital to:

- improve quality of life
- make life worth living
- develop a sense of belonging and being wanted.

All social contact may be avoided after bereavement, beyond that offered freely by close relatives and friends, who for many people can provide their only social involvement. This contact is often essential but much of this immediate support inevitably retreats after the funeral. Subsequently, it is important that people seek to replace the social void left by loss, with success often depending crucially on their willingness to utilise existing family and friendship support.

It is common for bereaved people to have a diminished interest in social functioning arising not just from grief, but from the disruption caused by losing a relationship which may have crucially defined a person's social role and emotional well-being. Important elements of social status, self-respect, pride, personal satisfaction, enjoyment and expectation may have been lost.

Old age itself does not necessarily make social reinvestment either different, or more difficult. Social relationships are in a continual state of formation, maintenance and change throughout life. There are many reasons why social reintegration may be difficult, depending upon:

- personal motivation and attitude towards a continuing social life
- cultural, social and familial attitudes about the role and importance of older people.

Some older people are often seen as a burden, whose life is coming to its end, and who should be content to tolerate their reduced social status and financial resources. Such attitudes, especially when accepted and internalised by older people, can be detrimental to how they adjust to loss.

However, some older people are not as active, and do not have the same social opportunities for replacing losses. Indeed, many long-established partners may have relied upon each other too much, becoming mutually dependent to the neglect of other social relationships. Reinvesting in new relationships and activities requires more effort than maintaining those which have become comfortable and easy through time.

For these reasons, older people can be vulnerable to isolation and loneliness. Some people choose to isolate themselves, perhaps as an expression of anger, grief, or hopelessness, thus giving rise to the kind of vicious circularity outlined in the diagram in Chapter 1. Degeneration into apathy, isolation, despair, and an unwillingness to continue living often results. The importance of hope is central to the task of caring for older bereaved people, particularly where this is conspicuously lacking. The counsellor needs to generate hope and optimism, and to encourage family and friends to do likewise. The central strategy in counteracting isolation is to encourage reinvestment in social life.

Offering bereaved people opportunities and openings for social support, encouraging the development of new relationships, and taking part in groups are central to full recovery. These can be achieved by helping people look at how they can reinvest in relationships. There are four immediate sources of support:

- to develop existing relationships with relatives and friends
- to form new relationships with other recently bereaved people, both to compare their experiences, and to form new outlets for companionship
- to identify established local groups of older people
- to identify established local groups involved in activities and interests shared by the individual.

Social activity after bereavement

The decision to reinvest in new social relationships is the ultimate indication of successful progression through the mourning process. But the counsellor needs to be aware of, and sensitive to the courage it requires for many older bereaved people to re-enter social life.

Bereaved people may find that their confidence in their social skills, and their reduced social and financial status, may be less favourable, and perhaps involve the stigma and discrimination of being a widow(er). There may also be altered relationship patterns, which may lead to family and friends being over-protective with older people, barring them from developing new activities and friends.

This process of social reintegration can be assisted by providing practical outlets for people which highlight not only avenues to personal fulfilment, but the positive contributions older people can make to specific areas of social life. One strategy, recommended by Staudacher (1988), is to set small, achievable personal challenges, involving simple activities which, when achieved, can lead to more difficult challenges being set as personal confidence increases. A positive circularity ensues which can help people re-establish feelings of personal power, and reduce anxiety.

Activity should seek to utilise and develop the interests of the individual, with the objective of enlarging their support systems. Many older people can be helped by an examination of their physical and social environment, listing the activities, hobbies and courses that might add interest and fulfilment to their lives.

> **General:** gardening, shopping, pets, sewing, knitting, crochet, reading, crosswords, jigsaws, travel, meditation, house redecoration
> **Start collections:** stamps, coins, scrapbooks, photo albums
> **Local groups:** luncheon club, bereavement groups
> **Further education/writing:** biography, short stories, life history, letters
> **Artistic pursuits:** drawing, painting, sculpture, photography, drama, reading plays, attending theatre, going to the cinema
> **Music:** playing an instrument, attending concerts, dancing
> **Sports:** walking, swimming.

Some people may find that pets can be helpful in supplying a presence within an otherwise empty home. However, in terms of conversation, socialising and human companionship pets are never a complete or total answer.

Loss is not always a negative experience. Some bereaved people discover that personal growth can arise, perhaps by moving away from earlier pursuits and discovering entirely new roles in areas in which there had been little previous interest or experience. The development of new skills, new abilities, and new strengths can arise, many of which were not previously required or recognised.

Some people may feel emancipated following the death of a long term partner, either through the freedom from the task of caring for an ill or disabled person, or the removal of an inhibiting or restrictive partner whose powerful expectations, or physical or moral repression, have impeded the fulfilment of the surviving partner.

Often, new social activity is connected with bereavement, involving perhaps particular aspects of caring, or fighting for the recognition and rights of particular groups, or charitable, social and political pressure groups associated with their experience of bereavement.

In these ways, the damage caused by loss to self-image can be repaired, and can often lead to enhanced enjoyment, satisfaction, fulfilment and expectation, all necessary for recovery, and a full life.

Companionship: the family

The companionship available within a lost relationship may have obscured the need for wider social contact so that after a significant death many older people can find themselves isolated and alone. There are many reasons for lack of companionship in old age after a major bereavement:

- lack of mobility
- poor health
- inadequate financial resources
- lack of confidence and self-esteem.

The rebuilding of self-esteem is best facilitated by social reintegration and the development of new relationships. Weiss (1976) outlines a number of needs that are normally met within relationships, all important when dealing with stressful situations:

- attachment to another person
- a sense of security, place, and being needed
- reassurance of personal worth and competence
- the availability of dependable assistance, advice and guidance.

The family often provides the most immediate source of support, and one which is often anxious to help. The family will have shared feelings and needs, and will have passed through the same stresses caused by loss. The family system is often distinguished by its common identity, its feeling of wholeness, the inter-relationships between its many parts, and the links it has with the wider community, society and culture.

Yet there are reasons why the family may sometimes be unable to offer support (see page 73). So whilst families may be supportive, some may themselves require outside help. One problem for older people concerns identifying a useful role within the family unit. Many older people do not want to interfere, or make any demands on their busy adult children. One major investment some older people can make is with their grand-children. This has the advantage of providing contact with younger people, which can be refreshing and stimulating, whilst also offering practical help to their parents. Yet there is also ample scope for tension and disagreement, particularly if they are seen to be 'interfering' with parental wishes.

For these reasons, many older people feel that they need to develop companionship and social contacts independent of the family, other outlets which are part of their own, rather than other people's lives.

Companionship: self-help groups

Group involvement can be helpful. Using groups moves away from the normal emphasis on one-to-one support, and can provide the basis for effective help. The initial reason for the group may be to focus on feelings of isolation and confusion, enabling people to see that they are not alone in their fears, and encouraging them to share their feelings.

Socially, groups can bring together lonely, distressed people to share their feelings and experience of grief amongst supportive people, dem-onstrating that the individual is not alone, and by comparing experiences placing personal problems into a wider perspective. Mutually support-ive relationships can develop within a caring group which can involve the individual in trusting relationships again.

Discussing grief with those who have survived can demonstrate that moving on towards a new life is possible, and can indicate that it can be done without belittling the memory of the deceased.

In recent years there has been an encouraging increase in the number of local self-help groups, consisting of formerly bereaved people, estab-lished to help people in mourning, particularly since the work of Silverman (1970, 1974). His 'Widow to Widow' programmes in the USA proved to be extremely valuable in providing counselling and practical support. Women who had passed successfully through the mourning process were recruited and trained to offer help and support to recently bereaved widows, with new widows invited to attend group meetings where they were able to meet people in similar situations, and during which a variety of grief-related matters were discussed.

The function of groups is to help motivate people to explore their worries and fears, and the reality of their present situation, and to assess how they could make better use of time left to them. Often, people attending groups pass through three stages, similar to those of the personal journey that has been described:

- the expression of confusion and anger, often complaining that other people cannot cope with their feelings and social isolation
- a period of indecision when individuals move from anger to a recognition of the fear, frustration and sadness of loss
- eventual acceptance, when individuals are able to look at the full impact of loss.

Many people who have moved successfully through bereavement decide that they wish to help others sharing the same experience; the 'helped' become 'helpers'. People with bereavement experience have been found to be particularly empathetic and understanding of other widows. The newly bereaved experience the relief that comes from sharing their distress and problems with someone who has a personal understanding of their feelings, and who has been successful in coping with, and surviving it:

- widows were perceived as being able to understand the conflicting feelings of grief, its pride, sorrow and confusion, rather than just offering sympathy
- widows were released from the constraint of worrying about whether their supporters would react with embarrassment and uncertainty
- widows could accept the normality of grief and its associated feelings, showing by their presence that life can still have meaning and purpose
- direct advice from widows can be more acceptable because of their status, and can provide encouragement to the newly widowed to help them develop new relationships and interests.

Others have found that formerly bereaved people can understand the feelings, and respond to the grief of the newly bereaved in a way which is both more appropriate and acceptable to those who need help. Schiff (1977), for example, argued that following the loss of her child more support could be gained from people who had suffered similar loss than from professional intervention.

Yet people may require help to identify groups, and encouragement to take part in them. They may feel isolated from the community in which they live, families may not know their neighbours, or they may perhaps come from a different cultural or social group. It is also likely that supportive networks may be absent, or even when they do exist, bereaved older people may lack confidence in making contact with them, and making new relationships.

CRUSE, the national organisation in Britain for bereaved people and their families, which provides a wide range of literature, advice, training courses for caring professions, and individual counselling, utilises support groups and networks, and should be able to assist in this way.

Diet and nutrition

Significant loss can cause a disturbance in appetite, both through over-eating (a substitute satisfaction) or under-eating. This can lead to weight change, and ultimately, damage to health. Many bereaved people, especially those living alone for the first time, stop preparing proper food for themselves. They neglect their diet, coming to rely increasingly on convenience food, eaten carelessly and haphazardly, and without regard to the effects on personal health. When people are distressed there is a tendency to eat carbohydrates and sugars, which whilst providing immediately satisfying foods, can be harmful to people with certain medical conditions. Healthy whole-foods, containing the necessary proteins, vitamins and minerals can be neglected.

Initially, this may be a normal reaction to loss. Bereaved people lose their appetite for weeks and even months, an understandable response to grief, depression and loneliness, and not usually a cause for significant concern. It is not vital to eat normally during such time, particularly if the individual is not physically active. Indeed, many people eat too much, and most modern health problems result from over-eating, or eating the wrong foods. Even loss of weight need not be significant, especially for people already overweight, and for whom weight-loss can be beneficial.

However, beyond this initial period, good diet is important if the possibility of illness arising from grief is to be avoided, and social activity encouraged. Poor nutrition results in people having less energy, and therefore less motivation to embark on activity. There is firm evidence that poor nutrition plays an important role both in causing illness, and contributing to the ageing process (for a more detailed consideration of the links between diet, health and activity in older age, see Scrutton (1992)).

Proper nutrition has to supply all the substances necessary for maintaining health, strength and energy, without making people overweight. The type of food eaten, and how much, are important factors in avoiding obesity, malnutrition, under-nutrition, and in maintaining the function of the immune system and preventing the risk of diet-related disease. There are four important principles:

- reduce fat consumption
- reduce consumption of refined carbohydrates, especially sugar
- increase dietary fibre (helpful in passing food quickly through the body)
- avoid food additives.

It should also be remembered that eating is a social, as well as a physiological function. Social eating is widely practised and enjoyed, but many older people find they eat alone, either by choice, circumstance or necessity. There is no reason why they should do so. Luncheon clubs are popular because of their social aspects rather than the food. Groups of older people can invite each other round for meals, supplying an excuse to cook, and an opportunity to share in the enjoyment of good food and companionship.

Exercise

Exercise can be an important element in recovery from bereavement. It is an important aid to physical, mental and emotional health. Physical fitness allows people to take more interest in social life, and enhances their ability to participate. Fitness involves several specific features, each providing older people with particular advantages:

- **Stamina** allows older people to do more things, go greater distances to visit and meet people, and to take part in more activities.
- **Suppleness** provides older people with freedom from pain and discomfort, with greater mobility and independence.
- **Strength** enables older people to continue doing more things for themselves and for other people, again increasing the sense of independence.

For many older people it takes determination to continue, and even more to recommence physical activity. Many social attitudes make us consider exercise and fitness to be unimportant for older people, suggesting that they do not need it, and even that it can be dangerous for their hearts, and injurious to their limbs.

This attitude can be particularly apparent in times of stress, including bereavement, when other people tend to take over many activities that older people would normally do for themselves. Consequently, older people can be increasingly denied the benefits of exercise. Again, for more information on the value of exercise in old age, see Scrutton (1992).

Relaxation and meditation

It is often assumed that relaxation consists merely of lying down and closing the eyes. In fact, it can, and perhaps should be more than this. In times of stress it is important for people to be able to relax their entire body, freeing it from its many tensions. Meditation is increasingly recommended for people suffering stress related diseases, particularly hypertension and heart disease, for it is known to lower blood pressure. Its value for relaxing the mind during times of mental anguish, and slowing down the over-activity of a troubled mind is being increasingly recognised.

The practice of meditation can be utilised during the mourning period, either individually or in groups. Meditation involves people in sitting quietly, with their eyes closed, in order to relax, to clear their minds, to ease, and to uplift (Tatelbaum, 1981). Its adherents believe that it can be a supportive, calming and relaxing experience, as well as an uplifting and moving one. There are many ways of creating this relaxation; one method is to concentrate on a simple, repetitive action, like our own breathing; another is to listen to quiet background music; another is to focus on relaxing the whole body, part by part.

Group meditation is usually preferred because of the social sharing, the physical contact of holding hands, and the powerful impact of shared thoughts that are believed to intensify the experience. There are many books on meditation, each giving a slightly different view on how it is best accomplished. It is well worth considering as a technique as an increasing number of people, including many older people, are finding it to be a deeply satisfying and consoling activity. As words can often seem so inadequate in offering condolences, meditation is another means of supporting bereaved people in their grief.

Artistic and creative pursuits

Many people do not find verbal communication an easy or effective means of expressing themselves, particularly in times of great sadness and despair. For such people even counselling can be difficult, and it is sometimes easier for them to express themselves through artistic pursuits. Clearly these have particular value to those who have lost elements of their speech.

Creative, non-verbal pursuits can be a method of expressing deeper feelings; self-expression is, after all, the source of most artistic inspiration. Drawing and painting, in times of bereavement, can express feelings that lay in the deeper recesses of the unconscious mind, and can often do so more effectively than many well-chosen words. It can be an important therapeutic tool for older people who are interested and skilled in artistic expression, although many people who have had no previous artistic experience can also express through art a depth of feeling that can be surprising, as well as valuable.

Tatelbaum (1981) describes a drawing exercise in which the individual is asked to draw whatever he/she wishes about death or dying arising from their personal experience, how they are experiencing loss, their view of death and dying, or a real or imaginary story about a dying, or dead person. When the drawing is finished it can be discussed to discover what can be seen.

Poetry is another useful means of enhancing recovery, and can have beneficial effects for several reasons:

- it may involve re-reading poetry which had significance in former times
- poetry can be meaningful to current feelings and cherished memories
- writing poetry can help express personal feelings.

Creative expression, whether through painting, drawing, sculpture, pottery, embroidery, weaving, woodwork, listening to music, playing musical instruments, writing prose or poetry, can all prove valuable for those people interested in doing so, and they can have longer-term value:

- they are satisfying activities in their own right
- there is satisfaction in creating something original, however small or insignificant it might be to the wider world.

The importance of creative activity is the value it has for the individual. What is created may never be seen, read, used or heard by anyone else; indeed, the individual may not wish anyone else to know what they are doing. The value lies in self-expression and personal enjoyment, not public acclaim. Even people who feel they have no creative skills can benefit. Further education classes can provide the opportunity to learn a few simple skills, and an incentive to start, regardless of age. Indeed, many older people have the advantage of both the time and opportunity, and recent bereavement may have increased both.

Returning to nature

Many older people find considerable satisfaction in direct contact with nature. It seems to provide some older people, who are themselves approaching death, and who may have recently experienced death close to them, some reassurance about the process of life, death and renewal. It can therefore have special healing properties for bereaved people, not least in older age.

Such activity can involve walks, bird watching, fishing, gardening, the collection of items such as shells, pebbles, rearing house-plants and herbs. Such pursuits have the additional advantages that they constitute good, healthy exercise, which is also enjoyable and relaxing.

6 Complicated reactions to bereavement

Blocked or delayed recovery

The bereavement experience is a natural, unavoidable, but essentially short-term reaction to loss. Recovery is normal, with the intensity of grief declining with time. Moreover, supporting older people through the experience is something that caring people have done, and will continue to do, through the ages.

Yet there has to be an inherent warning: the process of recovery can be more difficult. Whilst most people will visibly recover from bereavement within the first six months, it may be between one and two years that people fully recover from grief. Some people can become 'stuck', unable to cope with their feelings, or come to terms with their loss-diminished lives. The supporters of bereaved people need to be aware that recovery may not proceed normally, know how to respond sensitively to factors which may increase the vulnerability of bereaved people, and be able to identify signs of complicated reactions.

A few people may be so severely incapacitated they require more help than an untrained, non-professional carer can provide. When this is so, carers will want to be able to recognise the danger signs, and when they feel unable to cope alone to seek skilled assistance.

Yet it is dangerous to perceive recovery in terms of being 'successful' or 'unsuccessful', 'good' or 'bad', 'adaptive' or 'maladaptive', 'healthy' or 'sick'. The problem is how to decide, within the confines of individual experience, what constitutes recovery. The timescale and speed are hard to define, especially for older people.

It is normal for people to be unable to function adequately following significant loss, and it is reasonable that people receive more care, attention and sympathy during the grieving period. Yet how much, to what extent, and for how long this period of additional support should be is a more difficult judgement. The end-date of grief is probably less important than witnessing a steady, gradual process towards recovery, where – day-by-day, week-by-week – the individual can be seen to be improving.

Deciding when improvement is not happening is difficult. A single, reliable, universally applicable set of predictors would be helpful, but reality is more complicated, prediction more difficult. Indeed, given the variation of experience it is difficult not to agree with Parkes and Weiss (1983) that:

> '... most of these variations are within the range of normality ... that the pathological variations are no more than extreme forms that appear in response to particularly unfavourable circumstances.'

Complicated grief

Grief becomes 'complicated' when people feel that they cannot recover from loss, and when any amount of care and support seems unable to moderate their pain, or move them towards personal and social functioning. Horowitz (1980) has defined it as:

> 'the intensification of grief to the level where the person is overwhelmed, resorts to maladaptive behaviour, or remains interminably in the state of grief without progression of the mourning process towards completion.'

Chronic grief

Chronic grief is a prolonged, unremitting reaction to loss, where there is ongoing anxiety, tension, restlessness, insomnia, self-reproach and anger. It becomes clear that the individual is not coming to terms with grief, has become stuck, and has little apparent desire or ability to conclude their grief. Chronic grief can continue for months, even years, often with an on-going preoccupation with, and an idealisation of the deceased, a continued striving for reunion, a refusal to redefine personal goals, or to reinvest in future life.

Exaggerated grief

Exaggerated grief is an excessive response, an over-intensity of feeling, when people become disabled by an unreasonable level of anger, remorse, anxiety, hopelessness and despair, or when they continue to be totally or exclusively preoccupied with their loss.

Defined in this way, exaggerated grief describes symptoms which are features associated with 'normal' grief, different only to the degree to which they are manifested, when feelings of grief become overwhelming, debilitating, or lead to irrational behaviour. Whilst most people are able to test their feelings of grief against reality, some people, even with support and counselling, remain unable or unwilling to accept that their feelings are transient, that they can continue living, or that there can be meaning in future life.

Delayed grief

Delayed grief, sometimes called inhibited, suppressed or postponed grief, occurs when an individual initially shows little or no reaction, or one which is not proportionate to the loss incurred. For several weeks they may appear to behave quite normally. This can arise when important emotions are 'forbidden', or when someone decides not to deal with them during the critical early stages of loss. For instance, loss may occur when an individual wants to maintain social functioning in order to fulfil other vital tasks, or when they feel obliged to help other people.

For these reasons, people may decide to deal with their feelings at some future time, but by such delay they may cause a build-up of pain which can then erupt more intensely, more excessively later, when it may be more difficult to contain.

The initial absence of grief should be differentiated from the numbness and disbelief of normal grieving; delayed grief arises from a conscious effort to divert, postpone or deny the initial pain of grief.

Masked grief reactions

Grief becomes 'masked' when a person experiences intense emotional feelings, a variety of physical and medical symptoms, and manifests strange or untypical behaviour, all of which cause concern or difficulty, but where there is an inability to recognise that the symptoms are related to a failure to resolve grief.

Prediction: identifying delayed or blocked recovery

Carers need to be alert to circumstances where grieving is more likely to be prolonged or complicated, although again it is important to state that whilst these circumstances can more frequently lead to prolonged grief, they do not inevitably or necessarily do so.

All serious loss can have profound, debilitating effects. Grief is not a static, but a changing, shifting experience. Progress through the broad stages of grief, as outlined, may appear uniform, but it should be recognised that people do respond differently:

- some people are able to recover from loss without significant additional support

- other people overcome grief with the help of supportive relatives and friends
- a few people do not emerge successfully, becoming locked in complicated grief, seemingly unable, or perhaps unwilling, to recover.

The personal views, or fixed assumptions of carers about recovery should be avoided:

- 'She should be getting over that by now.'
- 'He is overreacting to what has happened.'

There is even a wide difference within the experience and behaviour of a single individual, who can swing from belief to disbelief, from recovery to regression. Conflicting feelings can operate concurrently in shifting, unpredictable patterns which can make it difficult to determine 'healthy' and 'unhealthy' responses to loss and poor recovery. Moods can swing rapidly from feelings of isolation, loneliness, despair, and a lack of desire for life, to sudden bursts of activity, an urge to recommence life and to plan for the future. This mirrors the twin desires of most bereaved people:

- a desperate wish to be free from the discomfort of grief
- the belief that such freedom may dishonour the dead.

In identifying poor recovery, carers should not focus on a particular day, but observe and analyse the progress (or lack of it) over a period of time. It is important to identify repeating and unchanging 'themes', or fixed outlooks on life, for it is these patterns which can signify a potential failure to recover.

There are some general guidelines that can be used to gauge how people are dealing with grief. First, some comparison can be made between present and pre-bereavement levels of functioning:

Recovering people demonstrate a progressive freedom from emotional pain, an ability to continue their lives, and to redefine their social roles, and an ability to enjoy themselves again.

Good signs

- The individual spends less time on negative thoughts and actions.

- The individual spends increasingly less time thinking about the deceased.

Bad signs

- The individual has an increasing tendency to dwell on negative thoughts; and may express self-destructive or suicidal thoughts.

- The individual continues to feel compelled to identify with the dead person in order to compensate for their loss; there are obsessive conversations about wanting to be with the loved one.

- The individual regains feelings of worth, disregarding feelings of personal blame.

- The individual resumes responsibility for self-help.

- The individual shows increasing signs of wanting social contact.

- The individual enjoys close relationships with other people, and seems interested in other activities.

- The individual enjoys a good state of health, or health recovers to its pre-bereavement state.

- The individual is increasingly able to talk about the deceased without significant emotional pain or despair.

- The individual is increasingly able to be happy in the company of other people.

- The individual is able to sleep normally, without bad dreams.

- The individual is increasingly free from grief, and is able to set tasks, and complete them.

- A sense of worthlessness and self-blame continues.

- An all-encompassing helplessness makes the individual dependent on others.

- The individual continues to refuse social invitations, makes no attempt to communicate and becomes progressively more isolated.

- The individual prefers to be remote, alone; does not want to be with other people; rejects chances to meet new people, or take part in other activities. The individual feels a burden on other people.

- The individual's health tends to be poorer than normal. The person develops physical symptoms similar to the deceased prior to death.

- The person cannot speak of the deceased without intense grief; avoids talking about the deceased, or mentioning the deceased's name; is emotionally affected when doing so.

- The individual is not able to laugh without feeling guilty. The person resents other people being happy.

- The individual suffers from insomnia, and often has nightmares.

- Relatively minor events can trigger intense grief. The individual continues to be apathetic, aimless; nothing appears to be of interest or value. Inertia sets in.

- The individual is in control of his temper.

- The individual eats and drinks normally and well; and maintains weight.

- The individual resumes normal activity, similar to the period before loss.

- The individual is less plagued with guilt and remorse.

- The individual gradually returns to their former self, both in terms of behaviour and personality.

- The individual's attitude towards the future is positive and realistic, displaying ability to think through problems with reasonable optimism and hope.

- The individual has re-entered social life as actively and effectively as prior to loss.

- The individual is able to look on death as a normal part of life.

- The individual displays overt anger and hostility with the least provocation.

- The individual eats badly, under- or over-eats, or abuses alcohol and drugs; and loses or increases weight.

- There is physical deterioration, lack of hygiene, grooming, or mobility.

- The individual continues to be plagued with guilt and remorse.

- The individual's personality has changed significantly; is generally more tense, discontented, withdrawn. There may be sudden personality changes.

- The individual refuses to think about or plan for the future, or to tackle problems in his or her life. There is continued pessimism.

- The individual refuses to re-enter into social relationships to the same extent as before.

- The individual has ongoing fantasies about death.

The gradual re-emergence of positive factors will indicate recovery. The continuing presence of negative factors should give rise to concern that there may be a problem preventing recovery.

The problem with such lists is that they outline factors common in all grieving. The difference between 'healthy' and 'abnormal' grieving is often a matter of timing and degree. There are responses which may suggest that the individual is failing to cope, quite erroneously. For instance, withdrawal from social functioning may be a 'positive' response of someone who wishes to deal with grief alone. Conversely, a person who engages in feverish activity may appear to be coping well, but their activity can be a method of blocking or denying pain, and can ultimately prevent recovery.

It has been suggested that eight factors are good predictors of recovery, as assessed after the initial four-week period (Parkes and Weiss, 1983). If several of the following dimensions, given in order of significance, are present at this time, the individual may find difficulty in recovering from bereavement:

1. An individual's own prediction of outcome

Those people most confident of recovering actually do so; those who feel they cannot tend not to do so.

2. The level of yearning

People who seldom, if ever, pine are likely to recover better the those who cannot take their mind off their loss, or who pine frequently, or constantly.

3. Attitude to personal death

People who would welcome death, or do not care about whether they die, are likely to face more difficulties than those who do not wish to die, and can look forward to life.

4. Duration of terminal illness

The more there is some pre-warning of loss, the more likely people are to recover fully.

5. Social class

The lower the social class, the more difficulties people may have in recovery. Several studies have shown that people with sparse resources find great difficulty in coping with the problems of loss.

6. Years of marriage

The longer the period of marriage, the more difficulties are faced in recovery.

7. The level of anger

People who express extreme or severe anger are more likely to face difficulties than those whose anger is moderate or mild.

8. The level of self-reproach

Extreme or severe levels of self-reproach give rise to more difficulties than when self-reproach is mild or moderate.

Factors relating to personal recovery

So why do some people recover from bereavement better than others? A number of predisposing factors may determine outcome:

> **but it is interesting to note that contrary to popular assumptions, most studies show that older people display less lasting emotional disturbance and deterioration in health than younger people.**

Given the pessimism that surrounds the combined experience of bereavement in old age, this is a significant finding.

Personality factors

The individual's inner resources are the most important factor in recovery. It is helpful for carers to know how bereaved people functioned prior to loss, and how they have responded to stressful periods in past life. Personal characteristics connected with high self-esteem are helpful in recovery, reducing the prospect of abnormal grieving:

- personal optimism and hopefulness
- resilience
- resourcefulness
- adaptability.

Conversely, a lack of confidence, an inability to tolerate emotional distress, and regular depression can make major loss particularly difficult to survive. Many will withdraw into themselves, their inability to cope with changed circumstances an added factor in their difficulty coping with life.

Everyone experiences change from birth to old age. Each move towards independence, from crawling to walking, from forming relationships to marriage, each change of home and employment, all require adaptation. Kübler-Ross (1970) called these the 'little deaths of life', and people develop strategies and behaviour patterns which form the basis for dealing with loss in later life:

> 'If we would face everyday changes, and practise letting go in our daily lives, perhaps loss and grief would be less traumatic. Even though we have a multitude of opportunities for learning how to handle grief, we usually avoid our feelings of loss. We bear up and force ourselves onward. Because we deny the full measure of our grief in our everyday changes and losses, when the big griefs come then grief feels unfamiliar, frightening, and overwhelming. Nonetheless, the death of one we love is so great and so final a loss that our past experiences with 'little deaths' may never adequately prepare us.' (Tatelbaum, 1981).

Older people do not usually develop new behaviours in the face of loss, although they can when it is necessary to do so. People rely upon the social behaviours and psychological resources which they have used before. Older people who have been resourceful in dealing with the vicissitudes of life will know from experience that they can cope, and recover. They will know how to respond, how to recognise their personal needs, how they can utilise support, and what they must do to help themselves.

Childhood experience

One explanation for poor recovery in later life is that its origins can be traced to childhood experience. Klein (1940) argued that adult mourning could be impaired by difficulties arising with weaning, believing that children mourned the loss of the breast. Bowlby (1960) supported this view, but believed that the principal trauma in children's life is the loss the mother, or the loss of her love. He thought that the origins of a depressive personality began at about six months, continuing into, and beyond four years.

Human growth and development consists of various tasks, the most essential occurring in early childhood. If the child does not complete these early tasks successfully, then his/her adaptation can be impaired in later life when trying to complete tasks on higher levels (Havighurst, 1953). Bowlby (1969), and Ainsworth and Wittig (1969) proposed that secure parental relationships provide the foundation for satisfying attachments in later life, a secure base from which to explore and experience life. The quality of these early relationships determines the child's subsequent capacity to make affectionate bonds. Erikson (1950) developed a concept of 'basic trust' which suggested that through good parenting the individual learns that he or she is able to cope, and worthy of receiving help when difficulties arise.

Yet whilst early secure attachments can provide the inner resources which help to manage stress in later life, inadequate parenting, anxious or tenuous attachments, can do the opposite. Young children who have not received consistent and secure parenting may, in later life, suffer feelings of inadequacy and insecurity in their relationships, and doubts about their ability to establish new ones.

Where a capacity to cope with loss has developed, people will be able to manage even the most extreme bereavements, at any age. However, where this is not present, grieving is more likely to become complicated.

The significance of loss

Attachment is both qualitative and quantitative, each loss relative. The severity depends upon a number of factors.

The length and duration of the relationship: the longer the relationship has endured, the more significant loss will tend to be.

Whilst age is not in itself a notable factor in bereavement, older people will tend to have longer relationships, thus often making loss more significant.

The intensity of the relationship: loss is more significant the greater the intensity of feelings and emotions.

This does not signify that for loss to be significant it has to be a close, loving relationship, as will be clear when ambivalent relationships are discussed.

The degree of inter-dependence in the relationship: the more dependence, the more significant the loss will be.

Although there is a tendency to believe that 'dependency' concerns one partner, two roles are required to form such a relationship. One partner must be seen to be 'strong' and 'able', the other 'weak' and 'less able'. Loss is significant to both; the former loses someone to look after; the latter loses someone to look after them.

The cause of loss

The impact of loss is closely related to its cause. Fashion has changed in this respect; in the ancient world, and within Nordic/Viking civilisation, a peaceful death was considered shameful, certainly for men, whilst violent death in combat was believed to be glorious. Current attitudes favour a more 'peaceful passage' where there is an absence of pain and suffering.

Discounting death in old age

Some deaths may seem 'more fitting', having 'more purpose' or 'meaning' than others. Some people may wish to die in a certain way, perhaps dying quietly in their sleep, in advancing age, or suddenly without pre-warning or pre-knowledge so that there is little time for fear. Others will prefer time to put their affairs in order, to make things right in their world, to say goodbyes. The fulfilment of these personal wishes may help survivors.

Loss in old age is often discounted, as is the pain and grief of older people, tolerated on the basis that an individual has 'had a good life', and that loss must be expected in old age. This can be a problem for older people: the experience of ageing does not alter the significance of loss.

Violent or mutilating death

Sudden, violent, mutilating death has become a potent reminder of human mortality and impotence, arousing feelings of shock, anxiety, distress, indignation and rage. The lack of warning can leave people feeling vulnerable and frightened. Identifying a mutilated corpse can lead to difficult grief, an experience which often needs to be discussed fully and openly.

Lingering or painful death

Witnessing a lingering, painful death through an incurable or wasting disease can also cause considerable emotional stress. The dying and bereaved live with death; it becomes part of their life. Yet when there seems to be no end to suffering, it can lead people to wish for death, or to feelings of relief when it occurs, thereby generating problems of guilt.

Cancer epitomises the long, lingering, painful death, with the unstoppable, destructive malignancy moving the body towards destruction. Moreover, conventional treatment for cancer – the mutilation of surgery, and the identity-changing side-effects of chemotherapy and radiotherapy – bring their own fears and distress.

Medical intervention

Medical intervention can exacerbate the problem with protracted technological attempts to save life, having a profound effect on both the dying and the bereaved. Intensive care seeks to prevent untimely deaths, but the tubes, drips, respirators and other machinery can distance and dehumanise the process of dying. Medicine also seeks to prevent timely, or inevitable deaths, prolonging the experience, raising false hopes, and confirming modern attitudes about the 'awfulness' and 'unnaturalness' of death. In these situations, medical considerations seem to take priority over the emotional and social needs of those involved in the drama.

Suicide

Suicide, where a person has chosen to desert those around them, is an act that leaves a devastating legacy:

> '... the person who commits suicide puts his psychological skeletons in the survivor's emotional closet – he sentences the survivor to deal with many negative feelings, and, more, to become obsessed with

thoughts regarding their own actual or possible role in having precipitated the suicidal act or having failed to abort it. It can be a heavy load,' (Cain, 1972).

Successful suicides often arise in families where difficult, ambivalent or hostile feelings already exist, and where threats and warnings have gone unheeded. Thus, suicide can exacerbate an already difficult situation, leading to 'corrosive' feelings which undermine the confidence of survivors.

Effective support should take into account all the social and family difficulties predating the suicide. Survivors often experience intense and volatile feelings, from shame and anger at someone killing themselves; to overwhelming sorrow that the person felt there was no solution other than suicide; to extreme stigma and guilt over the failure to see the signs, and prevent death:

- it can leave a sense of failure, impotence and abandonment, with intense anger when suicide is seen as personal rejection
- survivors can assume responsibility for what has happened, arousing feelings of guilt and shame about what could and should have been prevented
- some people may feel the need to be punished, often behaving so as to ensure that they are
- it can prevent carers responding, often leaving them with a sense of deep shock
- survivors can develop low self-esteem, based on a feeling that the deceased did not think enough of them to continue living, and that no one else cares.

It is often difficult to persuade people to talk to survivors about their feelings following a suicide. Religious disapproval, although less punitive in recent years, still emphasises the stigma attributed to survivors. Silence is therefore often reinforced.

Suicide is often considered an 'unspeakable loss', especially within families who may not want to discuss openly the circumstances of death. This can result in a conspiracy of silence which can harm survivors who may need to express their feelings.

There is often distorted thinking, where survivors wish to see the death not as suicide but as an accident, leading to the creation of family myths about what happened. If such myths are challenged it can lead to considerable anger.

Survivors will therefore often find it difficult to express their feelings, and they need to have 'permission' to do so.

Successful suicides are usually people who have not asked for help, whose signals of despair have been hidden, often because their carers have found it difficult to respond to their deep despair.

So there is no form of death after which discussion is more important. A common fear among suicide survivors is of their own self-destructive impulses, or feelings of fate or doom:

> 'They tend to feel more rootless than most, even in a notoriously rootless society. They are squeamishly incurious about the past, numbly certain about the future, to this grisly extent – they suspect they too will probably kill themselves,' (Cain, 1972).

There may also be support groups available, set up specifically for families and friends of those who commit suicide, which can be particularly important for people who do not have sufficient support from families and friends.

Sudden loss

Anticipated and unanticipated losses often have quite distinct impacts on survivors, with the trauma of sudden loss usually proving the more disabling, often leading to complicated grief reactions. These arise from the abrupt transformation of a stable, constant lifestyle into a new unpredictable, and frightening situation, where customary assumptions, ways of thinking, and behaviours, which have previously made sense of life have proved to be unreliable:

- security is replaced by anxiety
- assurance with disorganisation
- confidence with helplessness
- orderliness with powerlessness.

Parkes and Weiss (1983) found that recovery from anticipated and unanticipated bereavement took quite different courses:

- people who were told of an unexpected death, whilst understanding the information, were often unable to grasp its full implications immediately, and then entered into intense, deep grief which in many cases they stubbornly refused to relinquish
- people who were pre-warned of loss demonstrated an immediate increase in anxiety and tension, sometimes making an attempt to avoid accepting the situation; but this denial was not as severe, nor was their grief so persistent.

They concluded that the emotional reaction to the threat of loss is different to the emotional reaction to loss itself. Each is characterised by separation anxiety, the emotional urge to stay close to, or search for a lost person, but those who can anticipate death can learn to understand and accept the situation more easily than those faced with sudden death.

Ambivalent relationships

There is a tendency to believe that the loss of a close, loving relationship will produce the greatest grief reaction. This is not exclusively the case: the loss of ambivalent relationships also presents difficulties.

Most relationships are ambivalent, neither entirely positive nor entirely negative. This is true of many long-lasting relationships where attachment seems to have diminished, or been entirely lost.

Even within conflict-laden relationships, both partners can continue to feel attached to each other.

Ambivalence and hostility are not the same; ambivalence implies a mixture of love and hate, where attachment, however insecure, is part of the relationship. Ambivalence provides good reason for anger, often characterised by lack of trust, verbal and physical violence, and ultimately, conflict and divorce. One partner may wish the other harm, and when death or separation occurs the individual may believe, quite irrationally, that their wish contributed to the loss, leading to self-reproach and guilt.

The loss of an ambivalent relationship often follows a pattern. Initially there may be little apparent distress. There may have been scant affection in the relationship, and to express grief may seem hypocritical. Yet despite this apparent unconcern, grief can occur so long as there has been some meaningful interaction. In time, the relationship will be missed, the attempt to avoid grief will fail, and belatedly delayed grief may result. Even then it is often difficult for an individual to mourn, or to understand the conflicting feelings which can arise.

Many feel bewildered by their feelings when an acrimonious relationship ends. Why should they miss something they have not valued? Yet the loss of ambivalent relationships can often lead to self-punitive grief for several reasons:

- ambivalence, however uncomfortable, can become a way of living, with disagreement and dispute giving meaning and purpose to life
- tolerating an ambivalent relationship can signify an individual who feels unable to establish more satisfactory attachments, indicating a lack of self-esteem which can impede the formation of new social links, and successful recovery from bereavement
- conflict-filled relationships often lead to poor alliances with the partner's family, reducing the supportive network, and increasing those ready to blame them for the loss (Raphael, 1984).

It remains vital, therefore, to facilitate mourning following the loss of an ambivalent relationship by encouraging people to share their feelings, and to experience fully the pain of grief. This can help people absolve their feelings of guilt and self blame, their obligation to the dead, and enable them, through reality testing, to become more aware of what they have lost, to understand their loss, and to consider more creative ways of recovering.

Responding to complicated grief

Returning to the grieving tasks

Whatever the reasons for failing to recover from grief, it is important for carers to realise that people may require specialised medical or psychiatric support. Some people, however, can be assisted by those closest to them – and in any case, they will almost certainly require support in addition to any skilled input they may be given.

It is never too late to help bereaved people, however long in duration, or intense their pain may be. Complicated grief usually arises from the failure to complete one of the tasks of grieving, and the prerequisite for recovery remains:

the individual needs to be taken through these tasks.

Thus, if grieving becomes stuck, the aim should be to identify at which stage in the grieving process the individual requires help, and to help them proceed with, and complete the grieving process.

Task one: intellectual acceptance

There are many rational justifications for non-acceptance of loss. For instance, some people cling to the mourning role from which they may derive a sense of ongoing relationship with the deceased person, or seek to justify their continued helplessness. There is also the belief that grieving the loss of a genuine, loving relationship cannot, and should not end. Grief then fulfils another purpose: it becomes a 'monument' to the lost relationship, and everything it once represented. It is important to discover whether there may be better, more worthwhile 'monuments' – for example, continuing to respect their memory whilst honouring them through successful living.

If, for whatever reason, the fact of loss remains unacceptable it is important that the individual is helped to accept reality, to understand that they have to relinquish the past, and come to terms with their new life.

Task two: emotional acceptance

Unexpressed emotions, too painful to face, often lead people to preserve the intensity of their feelings in order to block other, more unacceptable feelings:

- an inability to come to terms with their former dependency

- avoiding assuming responsibilities for their lives
- a fear of the changes that are required to form new relationships and social outlets.

Where an individual cannot accept reality without painful emotions, help should focus on enabling him/her to feel safe about expressing feelings, both positive and negative.

One of key interventions in gaining emotional acceptance of loss is to try to redefine the individual's relationship with the deceased. The illusion of a continuing relationship enables some people to maintain a false sense of security, whereas recovery would necessitate giving this up, something which some find unacceptable.

Task three: adjusting to loss

In chronic grief, it should be recognised that:

anxiety about an uncertain future

is often as, and sometimes more important than

despair over a lost past.

Complicated grief can occur when people believe that the pain of continuing sorrow is more bearable, or at least more familiar, than the pain of adjusting to the future. Certainly, people who lack confidence in surviving alone may find more security clinging to a known, but obsolete world than facing the perceived problems and anxieties of the real world. To move away from grief exposes people to the uncertainties of a world in which they feel they cannot cope.

Yet in clinging to lost relationships people are inevitably faced regularly with their loss. Hence, their grief is endlessly denied and renewed. This is a particularly easy option for older people, for whom the future may appear to hold little attraction, and who may prefer to remain living in the past. Problem-solving has to be a major objective, where the individual is assisted in overcoming feelings of helplessness by testing new skills, developing new roles, and encouraging the individual to start a new life.

Task four: social reinvestment

The fear of new and unfamiliar people and situations can lead to social withdrawal, thereby removing bereaved people from the contacts that might offer the support and reassurance they require to recommence living. The chronic griever often lacks the confidence and security needed to foster social re-engagement.

Bereaved people are made to feel 'special' during mourning, when they are treated with gentleness and tolerance. In a perverse way, grief can bring a measure of attention and support – through visits, telephone calls, gifts, letters and other demonstrations of concern and sympathy – which many older people have not experienced for many years. Some find it difficult to relinquish such treatment, which can inadvertently encourage the continuation of grieving.

Unfortunately, people soon resume their normal lives, and expect bereaved people to do likewise. However, many older people, bereft of a significant relationship, can feel even more lonely when this happens. Some may learn that to be noticed requires a tragedy; they wish to prolong it, and accordingly they do not wish to return to normal life. So whilst direct support from friends and relatives is helpful in the early stages, as time passes there is a need to challenge people about the reasons for continuing grief.

People need help to free themselves from a disabling attachment to grief. Whilst continuing family and friendship links remain important, social support may need to arise from the cultivation of new relationships in new groups, and it may be that some people will require more support and encouragement to develop these.

Techniques of engagement, confrontation

Wherever an individual becomes stuck it is important they receive help to move on so that they can direct their energy towards recovery. This will sometimes involve confrontation. Certainly, any counsellor/supporter who remains content merely to facilitate the expression of grief may succeed only in colluding with self-damaging behaviour which can lock them in complicated grief.

It is necessary to promote the open expression of grief, but not sufficient. After time it is important to move on from being content to listen to expressions of sadness, anger, and guilt. Once these feelings have been discussed, the individual can come to terms with them, the blocks preventing progress can be removed, and progress towards recovery becomes possible. When this does not happen, the individual should be challenged about the reasons for their failure to come to terms with loss.

Timing is vital. Challenging is clearly inappropriate in the early days and weeks, but it can be done when it is clear that the individual is failing to recover over a significant period of months.

The method of challenging is important. Berating bereaved people is unhelpful at any stage, and is more symptomatic of carers who are not coping with their own feelings or frustrations than any genuine concern for the bereaved individual.

Challenging bereaved people should arise only as part of an ongoing process of caring and support, and a sincere unease that recovery is blocked.

Two factors are important when challenging someone 'stuck' in the grieving process:

- the language used should be direct and explicit
- there should be no compromise with, or pretence about reality.

One worry about challenging bereaved people is whether confronting them with the reality of their loss will increase their distress. The obvious response is that the individual is already distressed, and unable to move to any kind of resolution. Often the only alternative to challenge is collusion, a short-term attempt to keep distress 'within limits' by avoiding reminders of loss.

Termination

It is recognised in counselling that there should be a clear understanding between the counsellor and counsellee that the ultimate aim of the process is the achievement of autonomy. With formal professional arrangements this often takes the form of a contract. With informal arrangements it can be an understanding, regularly stressed, of the necessary limits to the commitment. The counselling contract, formal or informal, consists of two main dimensions:

- the duration – how long
- the intensity – how often.

The need to define these boundaries is mutual. The counselling relationship can be so supportive that an individual may rely too much on this alone, seeking to extend it into a long-term commitment as an alternative to attempting actively to rebuild their own lives. This can increase dependence rather than independence, thus defeating the ultimate counselling objective.

Dealing with specific behaviours

Self-neglect and self-harm

Self-inflicted harm may take many forms such as wrist-slashing, head-banging, biting or scratching. It is a means of:

- expressing despair and hopelessness
- allowing physical pain to provide some protection from the emotional pain of grief.

Too often carers do not understand these hidden messages, and respond with anger or incredulity, which can cause people to withdraw further, feel more hopeless, and less understood. There are no special techniques, beyond counselling the individual about the feelings which underlie their wish to hurt or damage themselves. Clearly, if someone remains intent on self-harm, more specialised help may be required.

Yet there are more subtle, less violent, sometimes unplanned, almost subliminal, but equally wilful ways of self-harm, brought about by an unwillingness to continue living. Despairing people, full of hopelessness, appear able to acquire, or give in to, specific illnesses – ulcers, cancer, heart trouble, nervous disorders – which can take over and even end life. The mechanism by which this is achieved remains uncertain, although it is believed to concern a relationship between the depressed mind and the body's immune system which in happier times is able to prevent such illness.

Suicidal thoughts

Bereaved people often experience considerable doubt about their abilities to cope with life, and an uncertainty about whether trying is worthwhile. So thoughts of suicide are not an unusual accompaniment to significant grief.

Suicide has many psychological roots. Certainly, old age and bereavement are two significant contributory factors. Suicidal thoughts accompany feelings of worthlessness and hopelessness, where there appears no other release from unbearable pain and despair. They serve many functions:

- a wish for reunion, a means of obtaining relief from the intolerable pain of separation
- the belief that it is impossible to continue living with overwhelming feelings of guilt, anger despair, low self-esteem, hopelessness, helplessness and powerlessness
- the feeling, common with older people, that life following major loss is meaningless, and death is an acceptable alternative to life without purpose
- a desire for self-punishment, arising from unexpressed guilt or anger turned inwards, a feeling that anger is best expressed through the 'revenge' of suicide
- considering suicide can seem comforting, a means of expressing intense despair, which may in turn lead to the belief that suicide is the best way of escaping it
- suicidal thoughts can arise from a feeling that no-one else can adequately understand their loss, and how they feel
- suicidal thoughts can help the individual consider, and come to terms with personal loss and death. If personal death can be tolerated, it can help them accept loss, making personal death less frightening.

None of these indicates a clear intention to take action. Unfortunately, there is no clear distinction between those people who consider taking their lives in the despair of the moment but take it no further, and those who are capable of doing so. Anyone capable of committing suicide has usually experienced substantial stress and fear, which can arise through the unbearable sadness of grief, a feeling that there is no alternative to their misery, and no prospect of rebuilding a satisfactory life for themselves.

However, in supporting people who may consider suicide, there is one overwhelming concern: the risk that they may actually carry it out. So it is important that carers are aware of the warning signs which have been found to be prevalent amongst those who commit suicide (Staudacher, 1988):

- withdrawn, remote behaviour
- perfectionism, with a high level of self-criticism
- depression, feelings of worthlessness
- frequent conversations about suicide
- a lack of energy, tiredness
- sudden, drastic changes in behaviour
- alcohol and drug abuse
- sudden disposal of possessions
- the writing of suicidal notes
- a sudden urge to put affairs in order, to change wills, to make arrangements for organ donation or funeral plans.

People who seriously contemplate suicide as a solution to their problems are often in such despair that the possibility of helping them is limited. Some people may appear unenthusiastic about seeking or accepting help. In such situations, it is important for carers to recognise their limitations, and to seek and encourage specialist help.

Carers should be aware of social disapproval, and develop non-judgemental, non-punitive attitudes to close friends and family. They should avoid reassurance, telling depressed people that:

'everything will be alright' and to 'look on the bright side'

or suggesting in other ways that their troubles are not as bad as they seem. Reassurance suggests disbelief, discounting the pain and depression that is felt. Distressed people seek understanding, and will often try to explain their pain. When they do so, they want their feelings to be acknowledged as genuine and real, and their pain treated as such.

Discussion of suicidal feelings is often considered a negative activity. It is not. It can help people through an excessive fear of death, and towards a healthier awareness and acceptance of death as a natural part of life. The ability to overcome personal fear of death can lead to a recognition of personal death. This can often provide the motivation for creating a fuller, more meaningful life NOW – for the recognition of death means that people can no longer take what life there is left for granted, and are more motivated to take action which enables them to live more fully. A counselling approach to loss should always inquire about the existence of suicidal thoughts. Worden (1982) suggests that to ask:

'Has it been so bad that you've thought of hurting yourself?'

is more likely to have positive results than to prompt someone to take self-destructive action. It is also helpful for the counsellor to 'reality test' the guilt, anger, shame and feelings of abandonment, and help correct any distortions about what has happened.

Euthanasia

When dealing with death, there is often an assumption that older people want to live. This is not always the case. It is common to find that many older people actually want to die, not as an emotional reaction to distress, but a thoughtful, considered judgement made on the quality of their life. They often wish to share these thoughts with carers, and very occasionally may ask for help or support in carrying out their wish to die.

It is a challenging situation for anyone to be faced with an older person who wants to die. Euthanasia is illegal, and contrary to dominant social and religious mores. Unfortunately, this does not resolve the issue facing many older bereaved people who have decided that life is no longer important to them.

There is a need to distinguish between those who 'wish to die' immediately after bereavement, and those who continue to do so after long and serious consideration. In the early stages of grief it can be considered a natural reaction which will pass. It is important, however, that such feelings are not discounted, and dismissed as a 'passing phase' which will decline given time. As with all expressions of despair and feelings of hopelessness, the wish to die needs to be accepted for what it is, discussed openly and honestly, and examined for the reasons that lay behind it.

When such feelings persist it is necessary to judge whether grieving has become 'stuck', or if the conclusion is one which the individual has reached after a careful consideration of personal circumstances. The difference is usually clear. In the former, the individual is talking from a position of despair and hopelessness, whilst in the latter, he or she is expressing a rational and considered point of view. Where this is so, there comes a time when it is not possible to continue arguing against what is a genuine expression of feeling by an individual about his or her own life, and its continuation.

7 Conclusion

Does grief ever end for older people who have suffered significant loss? The answer lies somewhere between yes – every individual can recommence their life, no matter how traumatic the loss, and how old they are – and no – it will never be forgotten, the gap will never be entirely replaced. The object should be to help older bereaved people move forward from the latter towards the former.

Working with bereaved older people is not an easy task. However, the rewards can be worth the emotional traumas that often have to be gone through. Many people have experienced the pleasure that arises from helping people emerge from their sadness, pain and despair, and begin living again. Recovery restores the capacity to have a full, enjoyable life, free from feelings of guilt, sorrow, or regret. It brings an ability to cope with personal emotions, and the problems encountered in continued life, accepting personal loss, and reinvesting in the life that remains. Thoughts of loss will often return, but they will involve an acceptable level of pain, and can be successfully incorporated into people's lives. Many bereaved people, particularly those who have received help themselves, wish to go on to help other people, to use their own experience for the benefit of others.

Then, maybe, this book will be helpful to them, too.

References

Ainsworth and Wittig (1969) Attachment and exploratory behaviour of one-year olds in a strange situation. In Foss, B. (ed.), *Determinants of infant behaviour*. Vol. 4. London: Methuen.

Bowen, M. (1978) *Family therapy in clinical practice*. New York: Aronson.

Bowlby, J. (1960) Separation anxiety. *International Journal of Psychoanalysis*, 41: 89–113.

Bowlby, J. (1969) *Attachment and loss*. Vol. 1, *Attachment*. New York: Basic Books.

Bowlby, J. (1980) *Attachment and loss*. Vol. 3, *Loss, sadness and depression*. New York: Basic Books.

Bowlby, J. and Parkes, C.M. (1970) Separation and loss. In Anthony, E.J. and Koupernik, C. (eds.), *The child in his family*. Vol. 1, *International Yearbook of Child Psychiatry and Allied Professions*. New York: John Wiley.

British Medical Association (1986) *All our tomorrows: growing old in Britain*. London: BMA

Brown, G.W. and Harris, T. (1978) *Social origins of depression: a study in psychiatric disorder in women*. London: Tavistock.

Cain (1972) *Survivors of suicide*. Springfield, Ill.: Thomas.

Cameron, J. and Parkes, C.M. (1983) Terminal care: evaluation of effects on surviving families of care before and after bereavement. *Postgraduate Medical Journal*, 59: 73–78.

Clayton, P.J., Desmarais, J.A. and Winokur, G. (1969) A study of normal bereavement. *American Journal of Psychiatry*, 125: 168–78.

Collick, E. (1986) *Through grief: the bereavement journey*. London: Darton, Longman & Todd.

Cummings, E. and Henry, W.E. (1961) *Growing old: the process of disengagement*. New York: Basic Books.

Dorpat, T.L. (1973) Suicide, loss and mourning. *Life-Threatening Behavior*, 3: 213–224.

Engel, G.L. (1961) Is grief a disease? *Psychosomatic Medicine,* 23: 18–22.

Erikson, E. (1950) *Childhood and society.* New York: Norton.

Freud, S. (1913) *Totem and taboo.* London: Hogarth.

Gorer, G. (1965) *Death, grief and mourning in contemporary Britain.* London: Cressett Press.

Havighurst, R. (1953) *Developmental tasks and education.* New York: Longman.

Horowitz, M.J. *et al.* (1980) Pathological grief and the activation of latent self-images. *American Journal of Psychiatry,* 137: 1157–1162.

Klein, M. (1940) Mourning and its relationship to manic-depressive states. *International Journal of Psychoanalysis,* 21: 125–53.

Koestenbaum, P. (1976) *Is there an answer to death?* London: Prentice Hall.

Kübler-Ross, E. (1970) *On death and dying.* London: Tavistock.

Lazare, A. (1979) Unresolved grief. In Lazare, A., *Outpatient psychiatry: diagnosis and treatment.* Baltimore: Williams & Wilkins.

Lendrum, S. and Syme, G. (1992) *Gift of tears: a practical approach to loss and bereavement counselling.* London: Tavistock/Routledge.
(Not referred to in text).

Lieberman, S. (1979) *Transgeneration family therapy.* London: Croom Helm.

Lifton, R.J. (1967) *Death in life: the survivors of Hiroshima.* New York: Random House.

Lindemann, C. (1944) The symptomatology and management of acute grief. *American Journal of Psychiatry,* 124: 1190–95.

Lorenz, K. (1963) *On aggression.* London: Methuen.

McEwan, E. (1990) *Age: the unrecognised discrimination: views to provoke a debate.* London: Age Concern England.

McNeill Taylor, L. (1983) *Living with loss: a book for the widowed.* London: Fontana.

Masson, H. (1984) *Applying family therapy: practical guide for social workers.* Oxford: Pergamon.

Mitford, J. (1963) *The American way of death.* London: Hutchinson.

Parkes, C.M. (1972) *Bereavement: studies of grief in adult life.* New York: International Universities Press.

Parkes, C.M. (1975) Psychosocial transitions: comparison between reactions to loss of a limb and loss of a spouse. *British Journal of Psychiatry,* 127: 204–10.

Parkes, C.M. (1981a) Bereavement counselling: does it work? *British Medical Journal,* 281: 3–6.

Parkes, C.M. (1981b) Evaluation of bereavement service. *Journal of Preventive Psychiatry*, 1: 179–88.

Parkes, C.M. and Weiss, R. (1983) *Recovery from bereavement*. New York: Basic Books.

Raphael, B. (1984) *The anatomy of bereavement: a handbook for the caring professions*. London: Hutchinson.

Rogers, C. (1984) *Client-centred therapy*. London: Constable.

Schiff (1977) *The bereaved parent*. New York: Crown.

Scrutton, S. (1989) *Counselling older people: a creative response to ageing*. London: Edward Arnold.

Scrutton, S. (1992) *Ageing, healthy and in control: the health of older people*. London: Chapman and Hall.

Silverman, P. (1970) The widow as caregiver: a program of preventive intervention with other widows. *Mental Hygiene*, 54: 540–7.

Silverman, P.R., MacKenzie, D., Pettipas, M. and Wilson, E. (1974) *Helping each other in widowhood*. New York: Health Sciences.

Simon (1979) *A time to grieve*. New York: Family Service Association.

Simonton, O., Matthews-Simonton, S. and James, C. (1986) *Getting well again: a step-by-step self-help guide to overcoming cancer for patients and their families*. London: Bantam.

Smith, C.R. (1982) *Social work with the dying and bereaved*. London: BASW/Macmillan.

Staudacher, C. (1988) *Beyond grief: a guide for recovering from the death of a loved one*. London: Souvenir Press.

Tatelbaum, J. (1981) *The courage to grieve: creative living, recovery and growth through grief*. London: Heinemann.

Treacher, A. and Carpenter, J. (1984) *Using family therapy: a guide for practitioners in different professional settings*. Oxford: Blackwell.

Weiss, R.S. (1976) The emotional impact of marital separation. *Journal of Social Issues*, 32: 135–145.

Whitaker, D. (1987) *Using groups to help people*. London: Routledge & Kegan Paul.

Worden, J.W. (1982) *Grief counselling and grief therapy*. London and New York: Tavistock.

Index